I0710832

Intermittent fasting 16/8:

The weight loss guide for men, women & over 50. *Learn step by step to detox & heal your body with this diet cookbook for beginners.* Prepare tasty & healthy recipes

Rihanna Johnson

Copyright © 2020 by **Rihanna Johnson**
All rights reserved

All rights reserved. No part of this publication may be reproduced or distributed in any form or by any means, electronic or mechanical, or stored in a database or retrieval system, without prior written permission from the publisher. The author is not a licensed practitioner, physician, or medical professional and offers no medical diagnoses, treatments, suggestions, or counseling. The information presented in this book has not been evaluated by the U.S. Food and Drug Administration. Medical suggestion from a licensed physician should be obtained before beginning or modifying any diet, exercise, or lifestyle program. The author/owner claims no responsibility for any loss, or damage caused or alleged to be caused directly or indirectly as a result of the use, application, or interpretation of the information presented in this book.

Table of Contents

Chapter one: Introduction to Intermittent Fasting

You look like millions of people who have tried different diets and wellness plans, low in calories, and high in carbohydrates, from an excessive calorie limit to 6 frequent meals. You found that despite all the promises and supposed 'evidence', everyone was equally ineffective like the previous one. Like so many people, you are probably tired of all the hype. The last thing you want to spend your time and energy on is a different diet! If so, this is great because I am not going to share a menu with you. This is not an entirely new invention of the fitness world and not yet another new hobby for health, based on crazy and unreasonable claims. Instead, it is the secret of weight loss, health, youth, vitality and longevity, which is based on ancient knowledge of how our body heals, regenerates and rejuvenates. This secret was known and used by significant figures from the past, from the ancient Greek physician Hippocrates to the warriors of Sparta and beyond. This is called intermittent fasting, and it will completely change your lifestyle, appearance, feelings and thoughts! Although long forgotten, it was recently rediscovered and quickly became one of the most popular ways to burn fat, stimulate your mind, heal your body, fight depression and give yourself the gift of a long life. First things first: what is intermittent fasting? Intermittent fasting (or ALS) is a term that describes how you can lose weight, your health, mind, improve mood and life through regular fasts and fasts off to change (often called 'feed'). People often confuse the intermittent position with a diet with limited calories. Still, although the IF gives you all the health benefits and weight loss during calorie restriction, it happens without overloading you a considerable thrust, crippling fatigue and a constant amount of calories that make up of a limited form of calorie intake. Another thing that distinguishes IF from other nutrition plans is that it is simply not a diet at all. Foods are challenging to follow, physically, mentally and emotionally stressed, and very often quite dull, limited and strict. The exact opposite is true; although you have to reduce your calorie intake drastically, this only happens for a short period. The rest of the time, you can eat as usual without worrying about grams, calories, and portions.

We had always experienced periods of abundant food supply, often followed by times when food was scarce, so our bodies are already cycling professionally between fasting and eating. Sometimes it's not just the skill with which our collection is designed to spend long periods without calories to consume, but also a great mechanism to achieve everything from weight loss to a longer life.

Fasting is not the unknown territory: Did you know that you are a seasoned faster? You can't see it, but every time you go to bed, you are practicing intermittent fasting, while sleeping! Every minute from the last meal at night to the first meal of the following day is a long period in which you do not eat, mainly a fasting period. The period from your first meal to the last meal on that day compensates for the feeding period. This is an excellent example of intermittent fasting principles. So if you usually dine around 9 p.m. and don't eat at 9 p.m. before breakfast, you're doing an impressive 12-hour fast without even thinking about it.

As you can see, intermittent fasting is not a radical and unknown new diet. This is the way we have always lived as a species. The only difference is that science is finally catching up. Clinical studies have shown that PHI is not just what you should do if you have no food or the ability to eat. Still, it is an essential part of maintaining health and maintaining your physical, mental and emotional state. While people have been fasting for thousands of years, trying to restore their body balance and revitalizing themselves, new studies show that intermittent fasting can be a cure for many evils associated with our hectic, overworked and malnourished modern lifestyle. It nourishes and is healthy. Now we have a lot of data to confirm what the old fast always knew: apart from sleeping, fasting can be the most critical, healing and restorative activity you can do for your body and mind.

Why fast? The benefits of intermittent fasting are almost too good to be true: If done correctly, you can do a lot of really amazing things in literally every part of yourself. When we say that intermittent fasting helps you, it sounds like a wish list for everyone's body and brain. The benefits of IF include lowering and controlling your blood sugar levels, helping you lose weight, lower cholesterol, give you unlimited energy, increase your brain power and even extend your life span. With such effects, it is not surprising that IF has recently become one of the most popular food movements. As more and more people see real results, they often lose the stubborn weight that they have carried for many years. Chronic diseases are destined to become even less important for life. Although this book is intended to show how IF looks, feels and operates in the following sections, let's look at the fantastic effects IF can have on your body, mind and life.

IF helps to burn body fat and lose weight seriously: it is probably more profit known intermittent fasting, and since most of the crowd of people rushing to this way of eating, trying to achieve weight loss is right that the IF, as shown, is an exceptional way to burn fat and regulate hormones during muscle building. And amazingly, this works much better than just calorie restriction!

IF change the way the cells, hormones and genes of your body work: who knew missing a meal could be so good? Every time someone practicing IF does not eat for an extended period, several exciting things begin to happen: they include cell repair, the balance of hormone levels such as insulin and activation of the protective genetic mechanisms that help them to become healthy and stay healthy longer. In short, the body takes the opportunity to make the necessary corrections and recalibrate itself.

IF can protect people from diabetes type 2, dramatically improve sensitivity to insulin and reduce insulin resistance: is a critical function can discontinuously after chronic cure diseases deadly in the world. Diabetes Type 2 has become too widespread. Because researchers now believe that the reason is to be found in the fact that, if we raise the level of sugar in our blood, so the calories consumed is higher than the needs of the physiological needs of our body. Fasting can be a much better way to eliminate diabetes and other medicines with traditional therapy.

IF can improve your brain: Yes, that's true. In many cultures around the world, limiting the amount of food you eat while studying is always considered a vital method to activate brain cells and improve memory. Now we know that this is what intermittent fasting does. We have always known that you do with your body what you do with your brain. Animal studies have shown us that if you have your ability to learn, remember and even regain your mood, YES is the right way.

IF is a robust inflammation calmer and can also put oxidative stress out of your body: If you ask each ageing expert to name two of the most significant factors in the ageing process, most likely, he or she will probably mention oxidative stress and inflammation. Both processes accelerate ageing, damage tissues and cells and cause unwanted chain reactions in body and mind. While these processes are an almost inevitable part of life, the good news is that interrupting fasting can prevent the worst consequences while at the same time improving your body's ability to cope with them, giving you a long time to look, feel and be run by young people. More time!

IF clears a backlog of damaged and dysfunctional material in your body: Each time we fast, it allows our cells to start the self-cleaning process, known as 'autophagy', which eliminates damaged and non-functional proteins and the accumulation of toxins. There are many indications that this process helps to prevent serious diseases, improves our overall system and keeps us fit.

IF has the skills of experienced heart healing: do you want to push away one of the greatest killers in the world? Well, intermittent fasting, even for a short period, is a great way to fight heart disease. Because of the ability to lower dangerously high triglyceride levels while increasing HDL cholesterol and a powerful anti-inflammatory effect, adding just a few days of intermittent fasting to your regular meal plan is a sure way to protect your cardiovascular health.

IF can be a cure for cancer which doctors have been searching for many years: intermittent fasting is so effective in reducing the risk of cancer and putting a body in the best possible position to stop the growth of uncontrolled cells. Researchers have asked the FDA to approve it as a recognized treatment for cancer. IF can also be the key to help patients deal with chemotherapy.

IF adds years to your useful life: with all the above benefits, it is not surprising that intermittent fasting has been found to help different living organisms extend their life and live beyond their useful life. But it doesn't stop there. Unlike other proven methods to increase life expectancy, IF has the ability to not only prolong your life but also to make you healthier, more vital and mentally better prepared, even in old age.

Do not eat at a buffet all day, and the post is not a hunger: Looking at the long list of benefits, it is hard to believe that something so simple, non--invasive and free treats and protects from much of the functions of your body and mind. That said, despite the IF being entirely blinded by the reputation of the majority of people, there is one thing that often prevents them from giving you one chance: part of the post. We were forced to believe that we could go anywhere and feel anything but hunger. The company's essential snacks and fast-food will already have given a bad name to appetite. With food advertisements that come across us everywhere, from the road to the internet, fasting seems too difficult. This is because we have been brainwashed to believe that if we miss just one of us, our body will be seriously damaged. However, of course, it is the exact opposite. We human beings are not and were not made to eat regularly all day, every day. Food is an incredibly complex and energy-intensive process, and every time you digest the menu, you use a combination of the brain, hormones, nerves, blood, internal bacteria and all organs of the digestive system. It is therefore not surprising that a short periodic break of constant feeding frees your body to recover, restores your energy, mood, the sharpness of mind and generally works wonders for your well-being. Don't get carried away by the myth that eating is often useful for your health. It doesn't matter if you plough through a bag of chips or munch a lot of cabbage if you overeat during the day, it will kill your body! Number one question I asked on those with whom I recommend intermittent fasting protocol is the "I" will not starve? "The truth is, that is, fasting does not starve!" This is an unpleasant experience, often painful. Fasting otherwise simply reduces food intake for a limited period. Those who exercise will tell you it feels great and will you also provide a list of incredible benefits. Genetically, we are always made to fast. To enable people the ability to spend a long time without built-in food, and when we do it, activate the root mechanisms, which help us to survive in these times, improve our physical and mental functions. To say that we always have a snack should take to be energetic and healthy, is not only wrong but also ignoring our long and very healthy food story among us as a species completely.

And most importantly, the restriction or seizure of food in terms of IF is temporary. I always tell cautious people that fasting is not eternal, but the effect is excellent. Once they understand this and start, they will never look back!

Who has benefited from intermittent fasting? Because fasting is an ingrained habit for people, and therefore, our body and mind are programmed to be able to *survive* not only during periods with low nutritional meals but to *thrive* and do better than when we usually eat. Intermittent fasting is an excellent treatment for weight loss and treatment therapy for almost everyone. However, there are a few notable exceptions to keep in mind.

Pregnancy and fasting: I never advise pregnant women to fast. This is because if you are pregnant, your body is already busy with vital and complex work. You support the growth of another being, and you really eat 'for two', so any stress disorder that can result from intermittent fasting is simply not a good idea during these nine difficult months. Although the tests so far have not been conclusive about the safety of fasting during pregnancy, I recommend that you make a mistake as a precaution and postpone fasting.

Diabetes and fasting: When it comes to people with chronic diseases such as diabetes, it is always essential to consult a doctor before you start a new diet plan. However, I would like to make a distinction here between type 1 diabetes and type 2 diabetes. Many people with type 2 diabetes have managed to control their condition and even treat it with carefully controlled intermittent fasting. Later in this book, I will provide scientific evidence about the positive effects of IF on diabetes. However, for type 1 diabetes, intermittent fasting is NOT recommended and can cause serious complications such as diabetic ketoacidosis. For this reason, I urge all people with diabetes to talk to their doctors about fasting before trying. Still, I also want to emphasize that it is not recommended to periodically interrupt people with type 1 diabetes unless your doctor asks you otherwise.

Growing and hungry children and adolescents: when the body is actively growing and developing, such as in childhood and early adulthood, it is vital that you support it by saturating it with various nutrients in large quantities. Moreover, since intermittent fasting actively changes hormonal production and secretion, it is not recommended for adolescents, as this may affect hormonal changes that are already taking place at this stage of their development. In addition to these exceptions, the vast majority of people are likely to benefit immensely from intermittent fasting.

And you have access to wonderful effects ranging from efficient fat burning and higher energy levels to a clear mind and a longer and healthier life. Every person who controls IF for himself discovers that it is positively affecting them as he never expected, so when you start this healing path, you will undoubtedly see that IF is recalibrating, restoring balance and healing your body and mind in ways that are not once mentioned. This is because the intermittent fasting - it is not a new and unfamiliar way to diet: it is your innate ability, built directly in your DNA as a human being. That's why, if you have any doubts about your ability to be supported, you will see how naturally and instinctively. In the next chapter, we will discuss the long and successful history of periodic fasting intermittently, and famous historical figures who used fasting as the best way for an active and healthy in mind and body repair that is full of vitality. And energy!

Chapter two: Intermittent Fasting: it is very straightforward

Intermittent fasting has become quite popular lately. But this is not new; it is even older than the ketogenic diet. Fasting is included as part of daily life in all cultures and religions. Historically, many associations with fasting are spiritual, but many also contain qualities that were beneficial for human health and seemed instinctive to be understood instinctively by ancient cultures.

The post is not new to any of us. Everything goes fast with us. From the moment we stop eating at night until we have breakfast the next day, we fast. The word 'breakfast' speaks for itself: from our first meal in the morning, we break our fast.

The only difference with intermittent fasting is that it is simply done with high intention. Instead of one window of 8 hours fast "by accident" during sleep, we deliberately raise it to a post of 12, 16, 18 hours or more.

There are various ways in which people practice fasting intermittently. It can be as simple as postponing the first meal to lunch every day, or as tricky as cyclically repeating different fasting periods at different times of the month, sometimes up to 24-72 hours or more.

Most of us probably grew up with the saying that "breakfast is the most important meal of the day." I know that I was. But it isn't. Postponing your first meal to later in the day is a great way to include intermittent control in your daily routine.

You may already be doing this unintentionally. I know that many people skip breakfast because they do not have time in their busy morning, or even because eating first thing in the morning doesn't agree with them. If it's you, you don't have to change anything! Don't worry if it's not you. It is much easier than you think.

Even our modern science supports the faith and practice of fasting the ancients. Studies show that fasting (among other things):

- Wards off chronic illness
- Lowers insulin levels
- Improves memory and brain function
- Improves cholesterol
- Reduces inflammation
- Increases our metabolism
- Increases energy levels

Intermittent fasting is also a powerful way to lose weight and not to regain it.

Although 12, 16 or 18 hours seems impossible without food, don't worry. It is important to remember that your body continues to receive all the necessary food and nutrition, but only for a shorter period.

Chapter three: 16/8 intermittent fasting method

This method, also known as the Leangains protocol, involves 14-16 hours of fasting with a feeding window of approximately 8 to 10 hours. This method is one of the simplest intermittent establish practices because after dinner (the last meal of the day), skip the next day, so you go almost 16 hours fasting. During a banquet, you can easily include two or more dishes such as lunch, snacks and dinner. For example, suppose your dinner ends before 8:30 PM. And don't have lunch until one p.m. From the next day I already hit 16.5 hours fasting between meals! While feeding, you can eat your lunch at 1:00 PM, snacks at 5:00 PM and then a hearty dinner at 8:30 PM and repeat the cycle. Although this 16-hour cycle is ideal for men, it is recommended that women do not fast for more than 14 or up to 15 hours. This is because many studies have shown that metabolism in women slows down after 15 hours of fasting, and instead of losing fat, they are starting to get it! This method can be complicated for people who are very hungry in the morning and cannot function without food. But instead of worrying about lack of food, you can consume non-nutritious drinks and lots of water to make your stomach think its "full", which reduces hunger. Moreover, it is better to keep yourself busy instead of messing around or doing nothing, as this can distract your attention. One of the most important things to keep in mind is that while eating, you should avoid all kinds of prepared foods and junk foods or foods that are high in calories. If you want to eat a bite or feel pain while fasting, drink two glasses of water and wait about 30 minutes. Your hunger will disappear. If you feel like eating sweets at the windows, don't look at cookies or chips or other food that is ready to eat. Instead look for something useful, such as carrots with yoghurt or cucumber sticks with hummus. This not only helps you to feel full but also does not add empty calories to your body! The best way to follow this intermittent fasting method is to combine it with a low-carbohydrate diet. Lack of carbohydrates helps reduce hunger and appetite and also helps to lose fat!

Just as every coin has two sides, nothing exciting or worthy can only be on one side. Despite all its advantages, intermittent fasting also has its disadvantages. Here we will see both the pros and cons of following an intermittent fast.

Chapter four: 16/8: The secret to losing weight is irresistible, health surprises and energy-intensive

If I could only recommend one thing to someone who is struggling with difficult or stubborn weight gain, is slow and suffers from one or more chronic diseases, these are these two numbers: 16/8. It's so! Why? Because these two small numbers represent a way of eating and living that is so revolutionary, so powerful and so simple that it would be unfair to call it a diet. Let me explain. How many times have you followed diets that promised incredible weight loss and vitality, but discovered that after a few weeks or months of reducing calories to a ridiculous level, the exercise is crazy, counting every gram and bite that enters your mouth? And, always obsessed with the right choice, have you climbed the scales and only seen the slightest weight loss? And how often have you noticed all those enormous vitalities that you thought you never feel like that might appear due to your new diet, you run out instead, excitable and always hungry feeling? If you are like most people, this is not an unknown experience at all. It is even so common that this is the reason why people no longer believe in diets. Well, I don't blame them. The fact is that a diet will never solve the problem of weight loss and health, simply because you have to eat, live, exercise and plan every bite in a completely unnatural and unstable way in almost all types of diet. Intermittent fasting method 16/8 is the exact opposite of a diet. This change cannot be everything you eat, count calories or not, you become obsessed with the amount of movement you need for your target reach. Instead, the simplest version of the 16/8 only requires that you make a small change: your schedule delivery. 16/8 in the name of the fact that you plan it 16 hours a day and fixed 8-hour feeding. Now I know what you think: 16-hour fast is no small change! I bet you believe this sounds worse than a diet, but believe me, this is one of the most straightforward and most intuitive movements you can make and make it a lot easier than you could imagine. This is because, although 16 hours sounds a lot, you will sleep at least 8 of the 16 hours of fasting. The so-called "16 hours" fast actually starts after your last meal at 8 p.m. or 9 p.m. and ends at 12 p.m. or one day of the following day when you have lunch as your first meal. We will cover the essence of the question about how the post 16/8 with to achieve success later in this chapter, but first I want to tell you why around 16/8 is effective method to lose weight and why my favorite type of intermittent fasting is for longevity, energy, clarity of mind and many other bonuses.

How does it work on 16/8?
The easiest way to answer this question is to say that it works intuitively. Why? Only because our bodies worked in this way before access to an infinite amount of food made us eat during the day. After that, we searched for food for a few hours, and by the time we had finished searching, cooking and eating, it was already noon. Because our ancestors never ate late at night, as we currently do, without thinking, your last meal the day before would, of course, be no later than 8 p.m. This means that after hunting and the next morning when they finally ate, they would spend at least 16 hours on an empty stomach. "Well, what then?" "This does not necessarily mean that the old form is correct." You see, two things have changed to stoically since the days of hunting and gathering. Humanity has never been so ill and overweight, and humanity has never been so burdened. Believe me; this is no coincidence. These two facts are certainly interrelated. Today we are told that we are always ready to eat 6 full meals a day! They tell us that our bodies need so much food to survive. But do you think our ancestors caressed coolers and prepared a bag of snacks with them in the desert? We don't even have to come back that way. Do you think that the generation of our great-grandmothers and grandfathers ran intermittently to eat six so-called "necessary" meals a day? The answer is absolutely no. And yet neither our old ancestors nor our great-grandfathers and great-grandmothers were overweight and did not suffer from the chronic inflammatory diseases that we have today. According to historical data, you will see that many people have not had breakfast in the past, but have eaten and dined early. Did they die? Can't they think clearly, live fully or achieve this? No, there is even reason to believe that eating less helps them to function better mentally, physically and even emotionally. Let's look at the difference between all-day grazing and breaks alone. Burning fat: Fat is the best fuel for our bodies. When you burn fat, you get a calm and stable energy source, which gives you many hours of vitality and strength. On the other hand, when you burn sugar, you get a quick burst of frenetic energy that

burns very quickly, making you more tired and sick than ever. Burning sugar leads to the accumulation of deadly toxins and the accumulation of dangerous diseases. Still, fat burning is a deep cleansing and eliminates accumulated acids and other unwanted substances. So, now that fat as the clear winner in the best fuel competition is established, let's talk about why our ancestors were able to burn fat and why it could not do effectively. Simply put, there's a whole day when we lose our ability to burn fat for energy. Instead, we simply store fat and burn sugar, which leads to weight gain and many health problems. When the body receives food every two hours, it does not have to dig deep and burn fat reserves for energy. Instead, the readily available fuel burns from food that it continues to feed. Usually, because it so often end up in a lot of food and do the kind of hard physical work that our ancestors did, the body will store excess energy the food itself as, you guessed it, FAT. Now we have a situation where the body is no longer burning their already large reserves of fat for energy production, but, as is often fed, it increases the reserves of fat! New York Academy of Sciences even published a report showing that consumption during the day has led to an increased risk of cardiovascular disease and stroke rates. And this is not just an assumption. There are facts for anyone interested in the search. Studies show that when people increase the amount of food they ate each day (even though they ate the same amount of calories) in just two decreased weeks, they lost a significant amount of weight, their energy, their cognitive abilities and their mood improved. They were also able to reduce their desire for food! Why did this happen? When they were about to spend more time between meals, their bodies changed from burning light and cheap sugar energy to regular meals to burning their fat stores. Suddenly these people lost weight without even resorting to reducing the number of calories which are consumed every day to bring their health and improve it dramatically by simple changes. This is the essence of 16/8: this is a change that will completely change your appearance, feelings and life. If you hold 16 hours between lunch and dinner, your body is free from digestion and metabolism, and you can concentrate on recovery and starting over. Facts show that those who fast with breaks when eating less food receive many benefits, including:

- Reduction of inflammation.
- Lowering of blood pressure and cholesterol.

• Improvement of the metabolism at the start of ketosis or the optimal condition for burning fat.
• Considerable weight loss that is easy to maintain.
• Prevention, improvement and even complete elimination of type 2 diabetes.
• Reduced blood sugar levels and increased insulin sensitivity.
• Strengthened heart.
• Removal of harmful visceral fat.
• Increased memory and learning capacity.
• Decreased depression and anxiety.

I recommend the 16/8 message because it is useful and at the same time, saturating, and you can continue to work and play as usual. But all types of intermittent fasting reduce oxidative stress, thereby reducing the accumulation of oxidative radicals in cells. This helps prevent oxidative damage to the proteins, nucleic acids and lipids of your cells. Because oxidative stress and loss play an essential role in ageing and illness, intermittent fasting is a powerful way to stop the tide of premature ageing and disease. Also, every time you get stuck, it causes a mild and beneficial response to cellular stress, helping your cells defend themselves against diseases and rapid ageing in the same way as with sports.

We recommend adding some practice to each fasting protocol that you use to get double benefits. I'll talk about this later in the book, so keep an eye on it. So, now that you are fully aware and accelerated to try your luck on a quick 16/8, let's see how you can do it. One day is typical in a fast 16/8 is so: you wake up and instead of cooking a meal, you take a coffee, tea or another drink - calories. Then, around noon, you sit down for a great meal. From this moment you can eat as usual until 8 p.m. when you should have been eating for the last time that day. You go to bed and sleep 8 hours and, of course, you eat nothing during this period. If you wake up in the morning and postpone your first meal until noon, you have just completed a 16-hour fast. Your feeding period is an 8-hour period in which you can eat freely, without counting a single calorie or without having to worry about a certain amount of exercise. You do not starve, you do not measure your food, and yet you lose more weight than you could even with the lowest calorie diet. It's as simple, and as a big fan of this IF form, I can tell you that I not only saw great results in others who tried that method 16/8, I never saw another way of eating that allows you to lose 4 pounds in less than a week without the usual torture that comes with diets! And the great thing about the 16/8 post method is that you can choose how often you want to do this per week. Some people start fasting only a few days a week this way, while others do it every second day of the week, and with ease, many people prefer to eat every day in the form of 16/8. The best part is the one which the schedule you choose, 16/8 one of my most IF to effective and people see real results much faster than they had expected. However, my recommendation is that even if you have to do it gradually, you have to work on making a daily meal plan for 16/8. This is because it often limits the time of feeding for 8 hours, the faster you will start to see the benefits of a surprise, which are practical for a reduction in blood sugar levels, increased mental clarity and concentration, and even better mood.

Unmasking the myth of breakfast: now I can almost hear the pants off the nutritionists stunned: "But what is breakfast, lunch the most important thing of the day?" Well, I will tell you a secret that can mean the difference between being overweight, unhealthy and tired or thin, fit and full of energy: NO BREAKFAST! Let me start by discrediting the old and tired myth that we have all been taught: ignore what they read on the back of the cereal box. Breakfast is not a necessary food, without which people simply cannot live. We do not feel very good at breakfast on a biological level, because it does not work with our physiological composition. Our body refuses to eat in the morning. I do not think so. Think about it: have you ever had a good and hearty breakfast that is recommended by many nutritionists, and then you felt hungry in just an hour or two? Do you not notice that in those days that you are late and miss the morning meal, you are less hungry and oddly less tired than usual? Well, this is not just your imagination, and of course, you are not alone. Breakfast activates the appetite and can keep us hungry and tired for the rest of the day!

Here is why: In the while, we have always been told that you have a place in the morning meal is the best way to get our day off to a good start, the truth is that this is the recipe for treating the disease, weight gain and fatigue. When we eat early in the morning, we mainly work against the natural processes of our body.

This may not seem like a particularly big problem until you realize that this high level of cortisol causes our bodies to secrete too much insulin when we consume any type of breakfast, even if it is a very healthy meal. When the load is released, insulin, blood glucose suddenly drops, making mood depletion grumpy and unstable and guessed it, a massive hunger attack. This does not happen in the same way at another time of the day, so a morning meal will not help us maintain a stable level of blood sugar to hunger, as we are erroneously told, often by experts. The research finally catches on with something that many people have been claiming for years. A recent study found that those who did not eat breakfast generally consumed fewer calories during the day than those who started their day with a morning meal. Other studies have shown that skipping breakfast with the 16/8 method causes a significant improvement in cholesterol, inflammatory markers and shows more weight loss than you would by merely calories to limiting.

This is huge: there could be more weight loss when transitioning to breakfast that is on a diet every day, even if you eat better food than you would if you were on a diet!

This shows that insulin control is one of the most important benefits of the 16/8 intermittent fast method. With the growing popularity of magazines on the rise, new results keep coming. So far, tests show, that missing breakfast can:
• Reduce hunger, limit cravings, and reduce the amount of food you eat
• Accelerate the fat breakdown
• Improve insulin and blood glucose stability.
• Stimulate the secretion of human growth hormone (HGH), leading to weight loss and better health.
• Protect your heart against diseases

From a personal point of view, after following many years of generally accepted rules and never skipping breakfast, I began to understand that both scientific research and mine and others have shown that it is very unhealthy. Now breakfast I do if I do not work very hard and I know I'm not in the food can fit if I do not. In the beginning, it was hard to get rid of the misconception that losing breakfast was probably the most damaging thing a person could do for his body and health, but after a few days without breakfast I felt light, energetic, and above all, I thought not that I craved more all day. Since then, I knew that I would not be forced to feed my body with a morning meal that I didn't even need. I know this will be a difficult step for many people because, in the end, we all became convinced that breakfast is somehow more important than any other meal. When it is difficult to find just your morning meal to give back, I recommend going gradually; there are smaller portions or delays in the scheduled breakfast for several hours. But I will say this: if you make a brave decision and miss breakfast for a few days, you will see results immediately. You will feel less hungry, you will be vital, and you will even notice some weight loss in the first few days. This is because your body no longer releases large amounts of insulin after breakfast to cope with this unnecessary morning meal. Once you see the incredible benefit of not forcing breakfast on your body when you don't need it, you'll never look back! I know that many people find it hard to get the energy they need to start their day, and many people see breakfast as a way to feed themselves in the morning. But the truth is that when you 'eat' carbohydrate-rich, starchy or heavy foods in the morning, you only raise your blood sugar and give you a feeling of incredible and ephemeral energy. After half an hour or hour, the daily reaction of cortisol naturally in your body, then rinsing with an overdose of insulin, will causing your blood sugar to drop and you will reduce energy. Going to breakfast for free does not mean that you have to do without fuel. This will be one of the main hacks IF will share with you; your look in the morning and your way of thinking, concentration and feelings in the early hours will completely change. And it is also super tasty! Are you ready? The secret is in coffee, not in old coffee: YES, it burns fat, increases metabolism, increases concentration and gives energy! This coffee is so effective, so plentiful and delicious that most people who replace their normal breakfast regret not knowing it before. So what's in this special coffee? To be honest, this is a straightforward and clean recipe. There is a mass-produced "health" drink, so you have to go buy it. You probably have everything you need to prepare this great cup of joy in your kitchen right now. All you need is a bit of good quality oil (preferably eating grass), cocoa butter, and coffee. Seriously, that's it! So what makes this the best way to replace breakfast? Well, first, vegetable oil contains common fats that are needed by the body to fight against bad cholesterol, and an excellent balance between omega-3 and omega-6 fatty acids, making it fantastic for the body's preparation to reduce the body's fat and if it was not enough, the combination of CLA and healthy fats, the production of ketones in the oil and coconut oil are intensive fighters against inflammation, which has been shown to reduce the fat mass, especially in overweight people. What about energy? Well, there is a reason why this coffee infusion replaced energy drinks for thousands of people with physical and healthy thinking (and almost all technological geniuses in Silicon Valley!). It contains essential fatty acids with a short chain, which increases energy levels and gives you mental clarity and concentration at up to 6 hours after a one-off cup! (If you want to try this coffee mix as a replacement for your regular big breakfast, I have added my special recipe to the recipe index, which you will find at the end of this book. Remember that you should not have more than a tiny cup during the fasting, however, because it contains more calories. If you feel too hungry or too tired to concentrate when you start to starve 16/8, this coffee is a great way to lighten your body after you don't eat breakfast) Nikola rather than violate his post, with carbohydrates! Now that we have had breakfast, I would like to say a few words about what I recommend about your other dishes. When it comes to food choices in version 16/8 of intermittent fasting, we say that this is not a diet, because it depends on what you eat during the 8-hour feeding period. Unlike other plans, it will not measure, count or repeat macros. However, having said this, I want to allow you to climb on my top slope to get the best results in the 16/8: take carbohydrate range. I don't want to say that you should not have any carbohydrates at all. I just want to say that when it comes to fasting for the first meal of the day, you should take something with protein and healthy fats, such as a good juicy steak and a few eggs on the farm, as well as a portion of low GI. Vegetables such as asparagus or spinach salad, instead of an option full of carbohydrates such as bread or white rice. This is because carbohydrates, as I will mention many times in this book, can quickly change many of the best benefits of your intermittent fast. One of the main reasons why the 16/8 intermittent fasting method works is that it controls insulin levels powerfully. Every time you eat carbohydrate-rich foods, you override this great benefit. Insulin is a hormone that accumulates fat and at the time when your body begins to take carbohydrates and metabolize, begins to produce the excess insulin. The easiest way to understand this is with this formula: more carbohydrates lead to more insulin, and more insulin leads to more weight gain, more hunger, higher blood pressure, faster ageing and a shorter lifespan. These effects - exactly what resolves intermittent fasting, therefore, to get the most out of your post, advise me that you never break the fast with a meal rich in carbohydrates and usually stick to a diet with low carbohydrate and high-fat foods during feeding. For the sake of complete revelation, I want you to know that many people fast 16/8 and eat a box of doughnuts during the feeding period. Many of them still lose weight because IF is so effective, but they don't lose how much they should lose and of course don't get all the stimulation effects in the brain that contribute to a long life and anti-ageing that you should get. I want him to get all the benefits of his job, not just a few pounds here and there, and I want him to sit down, work, and look great as he does this. Because studies have shown us that a low-carbohydrate diet gives you lower levels of insulin during fasting and feeding, this is the best possible way to get the loss of fat, energy, health and life you are looking for.

Does this mean that there are no carbohydrates? Not really. There are many good carbohydrates that I recommend including in your nutrition plans. While poor carbohydrates increase blood sugar levels and cause significant uptake of insulin, good carbohydrates do not raise blood sugar levels so quickly or so quickly. The best carbohydrates that you can add to your meals are not starchy vegetables. They are full of vitamins, minerals and phytochemicals, highly nutritious plant compounds, which keep you safe from inflammation, heart disease, ageing quickly, and even cancer. They also offer a large amount of fibre, so that everything is fine. This is especially important when intermittent fasting is performed because the lack of constant nutrition can initially make a person a little irregular. The fibre in vegetables will dissolve it quickly and naturally.

To help you choose, I created this list to excellently engage the carbohydrate during the portion of the diet that interrupted their fast:
• Artichokes
• Asparagus
• Broccoli
• Brussels sprouts
• Cabbage (all varieties are excellent)

- Cauliflower
- Celery
- Cucumber
- Eggplant
- Leek
- Lentils
- Beans (especially kidneys, chickpeas and green beans)
- Greens (including mustard vegetables, cabbage and cabbage)
- Mushrooms
- Okra
- Onions
- Pepper
- Radish
- Spinach
- Squash
- Swiss chard
- Tomato
- Watercress and all other green salads (including romaine, iceberg, chicory and arugula)
- Zucchini

When it comes to fruit, your best options are:
- Apples and pears
- Apricots
- Berries (including raspberries, blueberries, strawberries, black currants, currants, blueberries)
- Cherries
- Grapefruit
- Peaches
- Figs

My highest slope is for a more successful 16/8 plan:

Slope# 1: The example which I give here is based on my own 16/8 message schema, but it does not mean, which you need to dine at 8 pm the night before, and breaking the 12-hour fasting. This is how I do it, but you can have dinner the day before at 9 p.m. and fast the following day at 1 p.m., or you can have dinner at 7:45 p.m. and break the fast at 11:45 p.m. close to. Some people even extend their function from 16 hours to 18 or even 20 hours. They do this by eating the night before at 8 p.m., and then they eat nothing until 6 p.m. or 8 p.m. the next day.

This is an

extreme method that works for a small group of people and not one that I recommend because it is not possible for an 8-hour feeding interval, which, studies show, is one of the reasons why the fasting 16/8 works great. But it is really up to you how your body feels and your specific schedule. And of course, a message according to a somewhat modified plan is much more profitable than a word in general, because it cannot adapt to your day!

Slope# 2: Breakup With Breakfast For Good. The only drawback is that the program that you choose for yourself, for reasons of reason, must still prevent your breakfast (or morning meal that goes a few hours after waking up) from having associated with cortisol and insulin, which I explained above. You should also avoid having something to eat three hours before bedtime.

Slope# 3: For faster weight loss best rocket inflammatory effects, and improve brain functioning, and mood, the Target for high protein, high fat and low carbohydrate foods. As you now know, intermittent fasting in terms 16/8 is so effective, you can be crammed with carbohydrates in the feeding period, and you will probably still see pretty good results for weight loss because the fast mode makes your body go from burning glucose to burning your Madame marketing stocks. But, and this is great, but I would not use all the health benefits of intermittent fasting if I ate this way.   This is because a large number of carbohydrates, particularly simple carbohydrates, peaks in the causes of blood sugar, insulin triggers attacks and their inflammatory response is activated. It has now been shown that intermittent fasting works very effectively to cool the inflammation. Still, if it continually ignites the swelling that the pole is trying to disable, the swelling will eventually be applied. Regardless of how this way of fasting treats, if you continuously allow yourself to eat too many foods that cause disease, intermittent fasting in the world will not be very useful. That is why I strongly recommend that those who want to lose more weight, those with chronic diseases of any kind and type 2 diabetes, and those who need to see an improvement in brain function, mix this fast method. Usually low in carbohydrates. You could have the most carbohydrates to pick out vegetables with a low GI, no starch, and limited fruit. Also, feel free to eat as many tasty fats and proteins, as much as you want. If you are worried about getting hungry during periods of nutrition, remember that eating low-carb and high-fat foods give much more satisfaction than eating high-carb and low-fat foods. Think about it: if you are hungry, do you prefer: bagel or dried bacon, extra portions of butter and steak as big as you want?

Slope#4: when he is eating low carbohydrates, this has no relation to the calories or the control part of the slope related to the previous one. While the vast majority of people in Post 16/8 do it admirably and adhere to it, the few cases I saw where this did not happen amounted to one thing: counting calories and reducing portions. In short, if you convert this method of fasting into a low diet, where you have to start measuring, counting and worrying about everything you put in your mouth, you'll end up failing, just like any diet with few content calories. The reason that many people fast with the 16/8 method and see the latest results is that it is NOT a diet. Your 16-hour fast period is likely to last if you know that you are expecting enough food during the 8-hour feeding period. Your body will also understand that it nourishes and cares for, and will not attempt to accumulate unnecessary fat. If, on the other hand, you try to reduce calories and reduce portions drastically, two things will happen 1: your body will start fasting and adhere to a low-calorie diet, which is never a recommended combination. 2: Your willpower and enthusiasm will depend on all the usual things that make a diet impossible, such as counting, measuring and anxiety. The trick with IF is that it seems intuitive. When your fast is over, you eat real, whole, and thoroughly satisfying food until you are adequately fed. His body has decided to fast and organize a cyclical party, and he responds well to this type of food. Don't let the years of diet type come to mind and confuse. Listen to your body, and you will see these pounds slip away while they stay nourished, nourished, energetic and healthy. Join me in the next chapter to learn how a jerky post can eliminate one of the greatest killers of our time!

Chapter five: Advantages and Disadvantages of this fast flashing

Flexibility:
You are free to set or change your quick and bank hours as desired. It is not necessary that if you fast on Monday, Wednesday and Friday, you also need to fast on the same days of the following week. It doesn't matter when you're stuck, or you're stuck for a certain number of hours.

Leisure:
As soon as you start fasting, you will realize how much time you usually spend thinking and planning a meal. You will be surprised about the free time you have when you don't have to cook or eat every few hours. This free time can be spent on other, more productive activities. Many people find this freedom incredibly liberating.

Reduction of supermarket accounts:
If you skip one meal, you save a lot of money. Imagine not having to spend money on coffee or daily muffins (let's be honest, spend money on both!). Fasting even one day a week will significantly reduce your purchases.

Without complications, without expensive meal plans and comparisons:
It is not necessary for every bite you eat to keep, and it is not essential to compute the percentage or proportion of nutrients that you consume. You don't have to buy expensive ingredients or expensive food plans or advanced equipment. All you have to do is avoid processed foods, eat on schedule and only eat healthy foods. It's so easy!

Disadvantages of intermittent fasting

Difficulty:
People who are used to eating snacks or eating every few hours may find it very difficult to adjust to the long hours of fasting. Hunger pain can be uncomfortable, and in some cases, they can even be very painful also if they are avoided. In such situations, people usually give up and surrender to their itch.

Lethargy:
Although this is only a temporary symptom, inactivity is one of the worst side effects of intermittent fasting. Lethargy can be very difficult to work with and can cause some problems in your workplace. It would be better if you informed your direct supervisor of your change in diet and the associated symptoms.

Not stable:
Although intermittent fasting is beneficial, some methods are simply not sustainable in the long run. Imagine that you starve 24 hours 2 or more times a week. This seems impractical and such methods can only be used for a few months before the need arises to return to a more regular and sustainable cycle.

Chapter six: How to start

Intermittent fasting 16/8 is simple, safe and stable.
To start, select an eight-hour window and limit your food intake to this period.

Many people choose to eat between noon and 8 p.m. because this means that you only have to fast at night and skip breakfast, but you can still eat a balanced lunch and dinner, as well as a snack during the day.
Others prefer to eat between 9 a.m. and 5 p.m., giving ample time for a healthy breakfast around 9 a.m., a typical lunch around noon, and a light dinner or snacks 4 hours before fasting.

However, you can experiment and choose the period that best fits your schedule.

Regardless of when you eat, it is recommended to eat several small meals and snacks evenly throughout the day to stabilize blood sugar levels and control hunger.

To maximize the potential health benefits of your diet, it is also essential to stick to whole and nutritious foods and beverages during whole feeding periods.

Filling up with food that is rich in nutrients can help complete your diet and reap the benefits of this regime.
Try to balance every meal with a large selection of healthy foods such as:

- **Fruit:** apples, bananas, berries, oranges, peaches, pears, etc.
- **Vegetables:** broccoli, cauliflower, cucumbers, leafy green vegetables, tomatoes, etc.
- **Whole grain:** quinoa, rice, oats, barley, buckwheat, etc.
- **Healthy fats:** olive oil, avocado and coconut oil.
- **Sources of proteins:** meat, chicken, fish, legumes, eggs, nuts, seeds, etc.

Drinking non-nutritious drinks such as water and unsweetened tea and coffee, even on an empty stomach, can also help keep your appetite under control while maintaining hydration.
Overeating or overeating junk food, on the other hand, can eliminate the benefits of fasting and can cause more damage than good for your health.

Chapter seven: Intermittent fasting helps you reduce calories and lose weight

The main reason why intermittent fasting works to lose weight is that it enables you to eat fewer calories.
All different protocols include skipping meals during fasting. If you do not receive reimbursement by eating much more during periods of nutrition, you will consume fewer calories.

According to a recent study from 2014, intermittent fasting can lead to significant weight loss. In this review, intermittent fasting appeared to reduce body weight by 3-8% for 3-24 weeks.

When checking the weight loss coefficient, people lost about 0.55 pounds (0.25 kg) per week with intermittent fasting, but 1.65 pounds (0.75 kg) per week with alternating days.

People also lost 4 to 7% of their waist circumference, indicating that they lost abdominal fat.

These results are very impressive and show that intermittent fasting can be a useful tool to lose weight.

However, the benefits of intermittent fasting go far beyond weight loss. It also has many metabolic health benefits and can even help prevent chronic diseases and extend shelf life.

While counting calories is usually not necessary when performing intermittent fasting, weight loss is the result of the overall reduction in calorie consumption.

Studies that compare periodic fasting and constant calorie restriction show no differences in weight loss when calories are combined between groups.

Chapter eight: The benefits of intermittent fasting for men and women

The observation of periods of voluntary abstention from eating and drinking is relatively broad and can be applied in various ways. One of the things that cause fast blinking is remarkable is the fact that many people do not eat out - from hunger, but mainly due to routine. Intermittent fasting makes people more aware of food so that they quickly lose the habit of eating snacks, which often leads to poor health. Therefore, allocating time for several hours of fasting can automatically reduce the consumption of certain foods, resulting in subsequent loss of calories. Many people believe that the intermittent mode is convenient and easy to implement. The fact is that no specific products have, apart from controlling calories, this way of eating is ideal for many people. Several scientific studies have shown that counting calories and restricting the choice of food only makes the diet very much a task that can be stressful and more likely to lead to a rejection of the diet. It can also lead to a greater sense of deprivation, uncontrolled cravings, and even weight loss. It can be adapted to the intermittent post by a programmed manner of fasting and feeding, is solely based on time. Here are some of the advantages, which are associated with intermittent fasting.

Burner fat:

Intermittent fasting is an excellent way to burn fat, and by participating in fasting, the natural state of fasting in the body is generally extended. When a person is asleep, the body naturally goes into a state of starvation, where it automatically switches to fat-burning mode. When you wake up and start eating, the body starts producing insulin and releases hormone storage of fat, which then becomes a state of fasting. When you practice fasting intermittently, then you can extend the period of fasting for a while, and your body will continue to work in the fat-burning mode. Intermittent fasting also helps keep appetite under control. The human body is reasonably fit, and if you consistently skip breakfast in the morning, you will get excellent appetite control with less hunger over time. The body will find a mechanism in its way that allows for more efficient use of body fat and as an energy source. When the body burns fat as an energy source instead of glucose, the energy levels of the body will begin to stabilize and probably see hectic levels of energy all through the day, not with a sense of Kru savings of energy pulse. Because intermittent fasting leads to the burning of fat as an energy source; It also improves the body's ability to detox and recover. The digestive process usually requires a lot of energy and attention from the body. When you participate in fasting; It also gives your body to focus on other important things besides digestion, and which usually leads to an increase in hormone growth. The presence of growth hormones in the body helps in the following ways to improve healthy body composition:

- Keeps the body thin
- It increases the synthesis of tissue proteins, which help to promote the repair and recovery of muscle mass.

- Reduces fat accumulation.

- Strengthens bones.
- Improves blood circulation.
- Reduces symptoms associated with ageing.
- Reduces the accumulation of fat, among others.

Change the function of cells, hormones and genes:
Every time you run out of food for a certain period, different things happen in the body. For example, the body initiates cell repair processes, which are very important, and also causes changes in the hormonal level to make stored body fat more accessible. Some of the changes that occur during the fasting period include, blood insulin level is significantly reduced, which facilitates the burning of fat for energy.

Man of the growth hormone:
The level of the hormone on growth in the blood also adds to the level of a high, and these hormones as a rule facilitate the burning of fat and the gain of muscles, along with other benefits.

Cellular repair:
The body also causes significant cellular repair processes, which then aids the disposal of waste substances in the body cells.

Expression of the gene:
Also, the changes provided are useful in the molecules and genes which are associated with the lifetime and the protection of the body against diseases. Most of the benefits of intermittent fasting are usually related to changes in gene expression, hormones and cell function. When a person is hungry, the insulin level in the blood drops and also causes an increase in human growth hormones. Body cells also initiate essential processes like cellular repair and a change to enable the gene to work.

Weight loss and abdominal cavity:
Many of those who use intermittent fasting are usually motivated in favor of weight and body fat loss. With occasional fasting, you eat less, resulting in fewer calories. Intermittent fasting helps also improve endocrine function, which helps to reduce weight. A decrease in insulin level and an increase in hormones together with an increase in norepinephrine lead to the breakdown of fat in the body and also promote the use of fat for energy production. When it comes to dieting that leads to weight loss, most people prefer a diet that gives them more flexibility. Most people do not

like to think about food as it sometimes leads to loss of motivation after a while, to take part in limiting the consumption of calories. That is why many people prefer intermittent fasting as a way to lose weight because it is quite flexible. That is why fasting increases metabolism in the short term, and you can burn more calories. That is why intermittent fasting works in two ways to improve weight loss. This increases the metabolic rate by the distribution of calorie increasing and also reduces, which is consumed by reducing the food intake to the number of calories. According to the study, intermittent fasting over 3 to 24 weeks can cause a weight loss of 3 to 8%, which is a fairly large amount. There is the possibility of reducing the circumference of the waist 4-7% suppress the loss of fat in the abdominal cavity. This is a harmful fat, which is located in a hole of the abdominal cavity, and that is also a cause of illness. Another report says that intermittent fasting also causes less muscle loss than with constant calorie restriction. Thus intermittent fasting is a powerful weight-loss tool, which allows people to keep the weight loss over a long period.

Reduces insulin resistance and reduces the risk of type 2 diabetes:

Type 2 diabetes has become a common disease that many people experience. Typically, it is necessary for type 2 diabetes, as a rule, a high level of sugar in the blood relative to the resistance to insulin. Each power mode reduces insulin resistance may contribute significantly to reduce blood sugar levels. It then protects against type 2 diabetes, expressed by intermittent starvation to help adequately with resistance to insulin, which then leads to a reduction in blood sugar. According to several studies, the level of blood sugar in people with intermittent fasting are reduced by 3-6% in people who are hungry and insulin deficits reduced by 20 - 31%. Intermittent fasting also protects against kidney disease, which is a common complication in type 2 diabetes. Participating in a healthy diet, losing weight and exercising can be a great help in fighting type 2 diabetes. If you lose weight, your body becomes more sensitive to insulin, which at lower levels helps blood sugar. Intermittent fasting also helps those who are pre-diabetic, or even those with a history of diabetes in the family to remain in safety.

Reduces oxidative stress and inflammation of the body:

Oxidative stress is a condition associated with ageing and other chronic diseases. This is a condition in which unstable molecules, also known as free radicals, react with other essential molecules, such as proteins and DNA, and subsequently damage them. It has been found that intermittent fasting increases the body's ability to resist oxidative stress. Reducing the frequency of meals and calorie restriction can significantly help to expand the shelf for it due to increasing resistance to certain age conditions. Intermittent fasting helps improve the functioning of the cardiovascular system and the brain so that this, in turn, leads to a better useful life. Intermittent fasting also helps fight inflammation, which is another critical factor in all types of diseases.

Good for heart health:
Cardiovascular disease has been assessed as one of the leading causes of death, and most risk factors are associated with heart disease. Intermittent fasting helps to improve concerning the terms and conditions of these factors risk, such as blood pressure, triglycerides, inflammatory markers, and cholesterol, LDL and blood sugar levels. Intermittent fasting helps the body to a preserve circadian rhythm because it helps the metabolism. Having a healthy lifestyle is vital if one is to stay away from cardiovascular diseases. If you limit your calorie intake every day, this increases your risk of heart disease, insulin resistance and glycemic control. Keep in mind, however, that fasting does not mean a complete rejection of food; You can still have free low-calorie food, drinks and water.

This causes cell repair processes:
When a person gets sick, the body starts eliminating cellular waste, known as autophagy. The process involves the destruction of cells and the metabolism of dysfunctional and disrupted proteins, which usually accumulate in the cells for a while. An increased level of autophagy offers body protection against various diseases, including Alzheimer's and cancer. Starvation is activated via metabolism, which leads to the removal of materials from the waste material to those cells in the body.

Prevents cancer:
Cancer is a chronic disease that is usually characterized by uncontrolled cell growth. Because periodic fasting, as has been

shown, has a beneficial effect on metabolism, this leads to cancer prevention. Fasting also reduces those many side effects that are associated with chemotherapy.

Improves brain functionality:
What is good for the body is usually just as good for the brain. Intermittent fasting helps to improve metabolic characteristics that are suitable for brain health. Features include reduced oxidative stress; a decrease in inflammation, a reduction in blood sugar levels and a decrease in insulin resistance. It also increases the level of the brain hormone known as the neurotrophic factor. Hormone deficiency often leads to depression and other brain problems. Intermittent fasting improves brain health and increases the growth of new neurons, which usually protect the brain against any kind of damage.

Prevents Alzheimer's disease:
Alzheimer's disease is one of the most common neurodegenerative disorders in the world. Disease prevention is essential because no cure for this disease has been found. Intermittent fasting helps to slow its appearance but also decreases in the severity of in condition.

Life has improved favorably:
One of the essential benefits of intermittent fasting is the ability to extend your shelf life. Exercising occasional feelings has known benefits in metabolism and everything that contributes to longer life and much healthier living. Intermittent fasting causes the release of adaptive responses to cellular stress, which subsequently improves the ability to combat the disease and to cope with stress. Low-calorie diets usually exacerbate mitochondrial stress, which is useful in preventing ageing. The better mitochondria work, the better your body will work.

The science behind intermittent fasting:
We live in a modern age full of food, full of factories and agricultural or even food-like substances that have completely changed people's perception of daily food consumption. The diet has led to the many problems facing society today. While intermittent fasting is considered an old practice, the science underlying this practice has significant health benefits that people

understand. By participating in intermittent fasting, the body can repair itself, cleanse and even regenerate for optimal functioning in the body. As early as 1930, scientists began to study the benefits of reducing calorie intake by refusing to eat. The scientists then discovered that by cutting calories, mice could live considerably healthier and longer. According to some recent scientific studies, the same results have been found for different animals. Studies have also shown that a 30 or 40% decrease in calorie consumption, regardless of the method used, has helped to extend the shelf life by a third. It is also demonstrated that restricting food intake helps reduce the risk of common diseases. Fasting has also been shown to increase the body's ability to respond to insulin and also helps regulate blood sugar levels and control hunger. Different types of intermittent fasting usually have the same benefits, but different methods give different results for different people. Instead of forcing you to follow a specific way just because someone else has achieved your success, you must choose a way that makes you feel comfortable. Coercion can make the method not sustainable for you and that can only lead to the inability to implement it's benefits. Most food trends have their origins in science, although some facts are disrupted over time as they become popular. Once this diet plan has gained popularity, you realize that the benefits are exaggerated because the risks are also minimized. When demand turns a specific diet into a whim, meaning it becomes trendy, most doctors and nutritionists are more likely to exclude it, which can lead to a loss of benefit for their patients. There is a wide range of studies that confirm the many health benefits of intermittent fasting, although most studies have been done in animals, not in humans. It has been shown that starvation helps improve biomarkers of disease, maintaining learning and memory in the brain, and reduces oxidative stress and more. When focusing on intermittent detection, some of the common problems that scientists face are no longer comparable. What should you eat or how much should you eat? Focus shifts to when should one eat and whether he should eat at all for a specified period. Several scientific studies have shown that daily reduction of calorie intake is an effective way to lose weight and also helps to improve metabolism and cardiovascular health. People are always looking for more manageable ways they can use to improve their health, and many people are switching to intermittent fasting because they find it flexible. Participating in short periods of consuming a small amount or lack of food that contains energy is much easier to do.

Caloric restriction is one of the ways of dieting most scientifically established to aid in improving health. Some of the benefits of a calorie-restricted diet include improvements in the risk of conditions such as type 2 diabetes, cardiovascular disease and lowering cholesterol, blood pressure and triglycerides in the blood. Many people find an intermittent diet attractive because they can still lose weight with the diet and always enjoy the food they want regularly. A growing number of studies suggest that rapid blinking is one of the ways possible with a loss in weight.

Fasting and circadian biology:
Over the years, people have evolved enormously. In the process, they have developed circadian clocks that allow physiological processes in the body to function at an optimum level throughout the day. In CIRCA is this Dian- rhythm carried out after 24 hours light and dark cycles, the effect of changes in body behavior and biology. Food signals are usually the main temporary signal signals, depending on the daily rhythm, which then yurt provokes to the metabolic, physiological and behavioral pathways to regulate, which in turn contribute to the overall health and life of humans. This involves behavioral intervention because intermittent fasting helps to synchronize circadian rhythms. It also leads to improved fluctuations in the reprogramming of energy metabolism, gene expression and enhanced regulation of body weight and hormonal improvement. All these factors play such an essential role in ensuring optimal results in terms of health.

Microbes intestinal:
Most bodily functions are influenced by the circadian rhythm. The gastrointestinal tract, also known as the intestine, plays such an important role in the regulation of processes in the body. Many of the functions of the gut and other biochemical and physiological functions are influenced by the circadian rhythm. Intermittent fasting has a direct impact on the gut, thus helping to reduce permeable stress, reducing systemic inflammation and improving energy balance, which improves intestinal integrity.

Intermittent fasting has also been shown to reduce the incidence of things like lack of sleep, night feeding, and an increased risk of obesity, cardiovascular diseases and cancer. IF buoys lasting adaptive responses to stress, the cells in the body, which in turn the body copes with severe stressors that may occur, and ultimately the potential for protection against ill aggressions increase.

Chapter nine: Nutrition and dietary recommendations

Protein recommendations:
A common mistake when trying to lose weight is to overeat protein. As mentioned earlier, excess protein can be converted to glucose (sugar) and stored as glycogen. Due to the difference in atomic composition, glucose cannot be converted into proteins. Use the equations below to calculate your protein needs based on your goal. Weight loss = 0.36 g to 0.70 g per pound of bodyweight PURPOSE. Example: Mandy weighs 198 pounds, but has a target weight of 174 pounds. 0.36 x 174 = 62.64; 0.70 x 174 = 121.8 The ideal daily intake of Mandy's protein is 62 - 122 g. Mandy must now have at least 62 grams of protein per day to maintain muscle, but no more than 122 grams per day to prevent the conversion of protein into glucose. Bulk weight = 1.5 g to 2 g per pound of bodyweight PURPOSE. Example: John weighs 165 pounds, but has a target weight of 200 pounds.

Carbohydrate recommendations:
The calculation of carbohydrates can be complicated because it varies from person to person. Below are some guidelines that you can follow. Keto = 30 g or less per day. They must come primarily from green leaves. This method is a principle from a ketogenic diet. Plateau Destroyer = 100 g or less per day. This should mainly come from green leaves and resistant starches. This principle is useful when you have reached a plateau. Beginner = remove refined sugars. Rather than focusing on macros, a starting approach should be to eliminate refined sugar and take up resistant starches.

Eat saturated fat:

Fully hydrogenated fats become saturated fats. They do not contain trans fats. If it remains stable at average room temperature, it can be considered as saturated fat.

Examples of healthy fats:
- Avocado
- Fatty fish
- Olive oil
- Coconut oil
- Thick yoghurt
- Nuts
- Whole eggs
- Cheese

Cooking guide:
Saturated fat is the safest cooking ingredient. Unlike other fats and oils, fats do not saturate when exposed to heat.

Fruit Tips:
There is so much conflicting information about the fruit that they deserve special mention in this book. The simple fact is that fruit contains a lot of sugar. At the molecular level, your cells do not divide foods, such as fruit and chocolate, into ' healthy' and 'unhealthy' categories. Glucose is glucose, period. Any other form of sugar, fructose, dextrose and any other word ending with "bone" is converted to glucose and used accordingly. Fruit should only be consumed in season and tiny quantities if you are trying to lose weight. Our bodies are involved in the use of fruit as a loading medium in the cold months when there is not enough food. Our body is unaware that we live in a society where we have access to food all year round. And constantly eat fruit, talk to your body, that should move in a state store because the winter is coming. Here's how I recommend you use fruit when it comes to fruit smoothies to lose weight. Zanja consumes direct fruit after training with a protein shake. Never eat fruit without a protein source. Fruit smoothies are sugar bombs. The amount of sugar cancels out any antioxidant effect that the drink can have. Use green leaves to get the same benefits. Eating fruit after training with a protein shake is a great way to increase insulin so that muscle cells can absorb a protein shake. I know that the increase of insulin, as a rule, the red light, when fasting, to lose weight, but in this case, will help to increase muscle mass, because insulin also is responsible for assisting cells in absorbing proteins. If you want

to eat fruit as a snack, make sure you eat it with a protein source, such as nuts. This reduces the absorption of sugars into the bloodstream, gives it longer energy and prevents the loss of energy at the end of the day.

Breakfast rules:
Another problem that deserves special mention is breakfast. You have probably heard that breakfast is the most important meal of the day. This is true, but... You don't have to have breakfast in the morning. The word breakfast simply means fasting. Rest: fast. From now on, consider breakfast as your first meal, regardless of the time you eat it. For example, breakfast at 13:00 - 14:00. It is traditional for people more natural 16/8 to find this window to begin later that day to eat. This is not the gospel. Choose the window that suits you best. So if you are a person who hates eating in the morning, don't worry, this is not the reason why you can't lose weight. The most significant preference I can give you when it comes to your first meal is. Make sure it is high in protein and fat, but low in carbohydrates. The reason for this is that what you eat first determines how much fuel your body burns during the day. A carbohydrate-rich breakfast prepares your body for a search for sugar sources, leaving you with an unpleasant need for sugar, energy sauces and a cloudy brain. A breakfast full of protein and fat prepares your body for the search for fat as fuel and holds it longer. It has also been shown that starting the day with this type of breakfast helps with anxiety and depression, which increases the serotonin level. So ...

- Green leaf closed fruit smoothies
- Ditch grains for foods such as eggs and avocados
- Feel free to drop some grass to feed the mixture with meat.
- Avoid persistent starch in this food

Chapter ten: Exercise guide

The second visible piece of the puzzle is exercise. Exercise has many significant benefits. It can help with depression and anxiety, allowing you to achieve your aesthetic goals. Exercise also plays a role in the hormone balance mentioned above. Exercise promotes the production of growth hormone but also helps to deplete glycogen stores quickly.

Which exercise is best for fasting? It is generally believed that prolonged training of the cardiovascular system at a constant speed is the best way to burn fat. In my experience, this is not the case. Although it has its advantages when it comes to fat burning and ALS lifestyle, I have had much more success with HIIT training for female and male clients.

High-Intensity Interval Training (HIIT):
If fat burning is your mission, I recommend HIIT training. HIIT can be performed with exercises with bodyweight, kettlebell, and dumbbells. I usually look for exercises that use more than one muscle group. The name of the game is short bursts with almost maximum effort. Here are some guidelines you can play with.

➢ 20 seconds of exercise - 10 seconds of rest (advanced)
➢ 10 seconds of training - 20 seconds rest (average)
➢ 10 seconds exercise - 30 seconds rest (for beginners)

You complete:
➢ 8+ (advanced)
➢ 3-6 (average)
➢ 1-3 (beginner)

The number of exercises:
➢ 7+ (advanced)
➢ 5-6 (average)
➢ 3-5 (beginner)

Training examples

Novice:
➢ Squats
➢ Run on-site
➢ Star Jump

Intermediate:
➢ Burpees

➢ Weighted squat
➢ Click on Up
➢ Medicinal ball
➢ Fight ropes

Also:
➢ Burpee / high jump
➢ Boxing jump
➢ Kettlebell swing
➢ Clean and press
➢ Fight ropes
➢ Kettlebell Row

Chapter eleven: Breakfast Recipes

❖ Boiled eggs and bacon on toast:

The soft bacon crispy in the pan is the perfect start for every morning. Imagine that fleshy and tasty scent that stays in the air, even if it is in the stomach; How can you get hungry afterwards? Make your breakfast more plentiful by covering the toast with eggs, and you never have to worry about growling in the middle of the 11 am meeting.

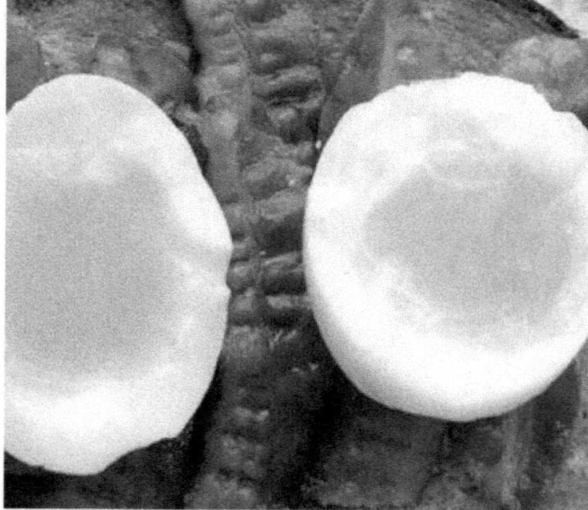

Preparation time: 5 minutes

Preparation time: 15 minutes.

Ingredients:
- two slices of bacon
- two medium eggs
- 200 grams of spinach leaf
- salmon (optional)
- one slice of toast
- sea salt
- slack pepper

Instructions:

1. Place a large pan with water on low heat.
2. Gently shake the water and break the eggs; cook for 4 minutes or until the white is ready.
3. Meanwhile, heat a frying pan, add some water and add spinach. Bake for 2 minutes until it has wilted.
4. Remove the spinach and place on a plate. Bake the bacon until golden brown.
5. Put spinach (and salmon) on toast, salt and pepper.
6. Cover if all were poached eggs and bacon.

NUTRITIONAL INFORMATION:
356 calories 23 grams of fat Total 15 g of carbohydrates 0.77 g of pure carbohydrates | 0.2 g of fibre 26 g of protein

❖ **Cinnamon buns:**

There is nothing better than starting the day with the cozy aroma of cinnamon and freshly baked bread. As the name suggests, these sturdy cinnamon buns are incredibly soft, chewy and sweet.

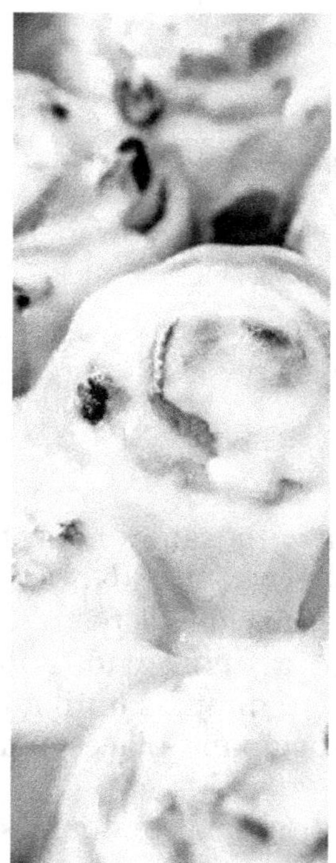

Preparation time: 45 minutes, plus an hour and 45 minutes for the dough to rise

Preparation time: 20 minutes.

Creates: 24 rolls

Ingredients:
- 1 cup whole meal flour
- 3 cups all-purpose flour
- Active-active dry yeast
- 1 cup of soy milk or milk
- ¾ cup of sugar
- ¼ cup of vegetable oil
- 1 teaspoon of salt
- four proteins
- ¼ cup of trans-fat-free margarine
- two teaspoons of cinnamon
- 1 cup of powdered sugar
- ½ teaspoon of pure vanilla extract
- two tablespoons of soy milk or milk

Instructions:

1. Combine whole meal flour, 1 cup of all-purpose flour and yeast in a large bowl. Set aside.
2. Combine soy milk, ¼ cup of sugar, butter and salt in a saucepan and simmer until hot. Stir to mix and then add to the flour and yeast mixture. Beat the egg whites.
3. Hit at high speed for about 4 minutes and regularly stop to scrape on the sides.
4. Add most of the remaining flour to make one enormously hard.
5. Remove the dough from a bowl and place it on a floured surface. Knead the dough for 10 minutes and if necessary add more flour to a tablespoon to prevent sticking.
6. Place the dough in a greased bowl and then turn to grease the top of the bowl. Cover with a towel and let it grow in a warm place until it doubles (about an hour).
7. Beat the dough and divide it into two parts. Roll each piece of dough in a rectangle thickness of approximately ¼ inch.

8. Melt the margarine and peel it over the rectangle of the dough. Mix in a small cup of cinnamon and the remaining half cup of sugar and divide the mixture evenly over both squares of the dough.
9. Fold the rectangles starting at the most extensive ends. Pinch the ends with your fingers and press the seams into the mixture.
10. Cut the rollers in pieces of 1 - inch and put the pieces into a greased baking tray two plates or round shapes non-stick 9 inches. Cover each dish with a towel or waxed paper and let the rolls rise in a warm place until they double (about 45 minutes). Preheat the oven to 375 degrees.

11. Bake for 20 minutes.
12. While the muffins are baking, prepare the icing by mixing powdered sugar, vanilla and one tablespoon of soy milk. Add extra soy milk in 1 teaspoon increments until the frosting is thick but spilt. Spray ice on warm rolls; to enjoy.

NUTRITIONAL INFORMATION:

243 calories | 9 grams of fat Total carbohydrate 15 g | 1.4 g of fibre 4.2 g of protein

❖ **Avocado burger with chilli and beef :**

This can be our favorite! Also, if you are concerned about practicing intermittent fasting, while still a diet of fat, this recipe can be made by dropping the bread; You do not have to give up one after the other. And here is an example of how you can reap the health benefits of both diets in one dish!

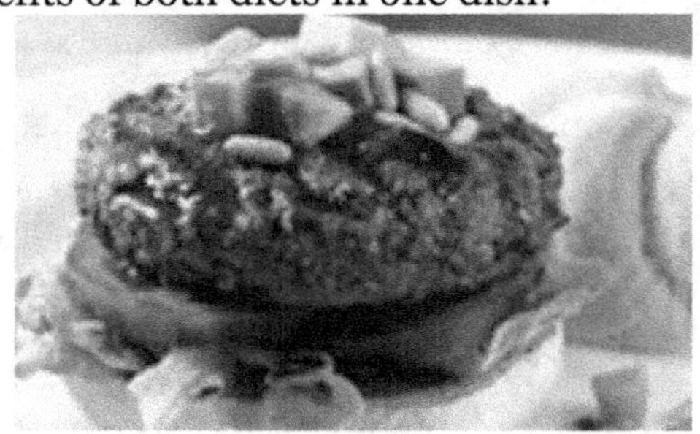

Preparation time: 15 minutes

Preparation time: 10 minutes.

Makes: 2 Hamburgers

Ingredients:

- 400 glean meat
- 2 red chilli peppers
- Burger Bun (optional)
- Sea salt
- Black pepper
- one medium-sized ripe avocado
- two dried tomatoes
- one lemon juice

Instructions:

1. Combine the meat and half of the chopped jalapeno in a bowl, season with salt and pepper and divide into four balls. Flatten them all and set them aside.
2. Cut the avocado in two, take the meat in a bowl and crush it with a fork.

3. Add the remaining chili peppers, dried tomatoes and lemon juice with pureed avocado.
4. Place a tablespoon of avocado mixture in the middle of the two empanadas and cover each with the remaining empanadas. Click on the edges to close the avocado in the middle of the hamburger.
5. Heat the pan over high heat, add the burgers and bake for 5 minutes on each side until they are well done.
6. If you decide to use sandwiches, place the cooked avocado patties between two sandwiches (you can only use one if you want to reduce the number of calories). Consider using whole-grain bread to feel full longer.

NUTRITIONAL INFORMATION:
1030 calories 70 grams of fat 51 g total carbohydrates 1.4 g of fibre 52 g of protein

❖ **Cajun red beans and rice:**

If the idea of spending hours in the kitchen scares you, you'll appreciate the uncomplicated nature of this dish. If you cook rice in advance, you will find that this traditional American dish on the south coast needs very little time to prepare.

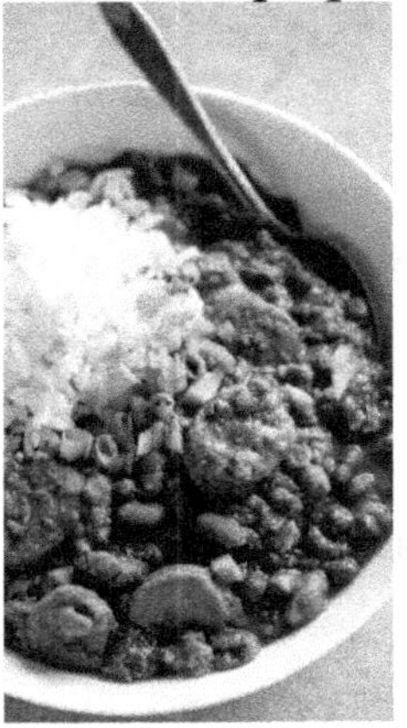

Preparation time: 10 minutes

Preparation time: 15 minutes.

Output: 8 portions

Ingredients:

- three tablespoons olive oil
- one large onion, minced
- 3 finely chopped garlic cloves
- ½ cup chopped green pepper
- one celery stem, including green leaves, finely chopped
- ½ teaspoon of salt
- 1 teaspoon caraway seeds
- 1 tablespoon chilli powder
- ½ teaspoon of thyme
- Two cans of 15 grams of dark red beans, rinsed and dried
- 20½ cups of cooked rice
- Fresh parsley for decoration

Instructions:

1. Heat the olive oil in a large pan. Cook the onions, garlic, bell pepper and celery in oil over medium heat until the onions become clear (about 7 minutes). Add salt, cumin, chilli powder and thyme. Shake to combine.
2. Add the beans and mix well. Reduce the heat to a minimum and continue to cook for a few minutes until the beans are hot. Make sure you stir regularly to prevent sticking.
3. Add rice to the bean mixture and mix all ingredients well. Cook for about 5 minutes to heat rice before serving.

NUTRITIONAL INFORMATION:

112.9 g calories 2.6 g fat 18 g total carbohydrates 6.4 g of fibre 5.1 g of protein

❖ **Keto waffles**

Preparation time 10 minutes

Preparation time 20 minutes

Total time: 30 minutes.

Servings per package: 5

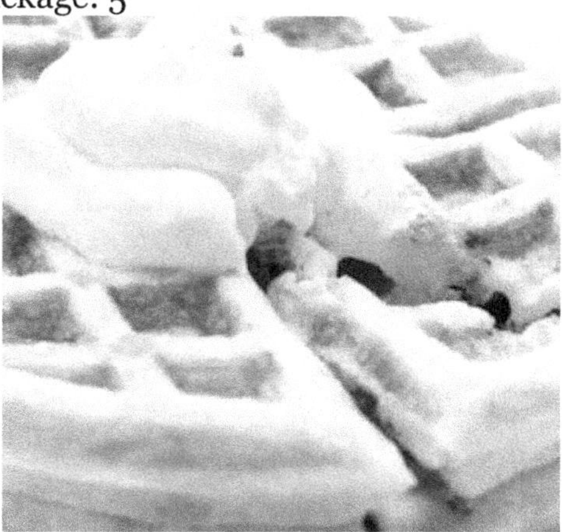

Ingredients:

- five eggs - individual
- four tablespoons almond flour
- one teaspoon of stevia
- one teaspoon of baking powder
- two teaspoons vanilla
- three tablespoons whipped cream
- 125 g unsalted butter, melted

Instructions:

1. Preheat the kettle/cookie according to the manufacturer's instructions.
2. Beat the egg whites in a small bowl with an electric mixer until they harden and form hard spikes.
3. In a second bowl, combine egg yolks, almond flour, stevia and baking powder.
4. Slowly add the melted butter to the egg yolk mixture.
5. Add cream and vanilla and mix well.
6. Carefully add the egg whites to the egg yolk mixture and mix.
7. Pour two tablespoons. Waffles mixture in a pre-heated waffle iron. Bake on both sides until golden brown.

8. Store hot waffles in a preheated oven in the lowest position.
9. Repeat this until all the mixture has been used.
10. Serve with butter or another keto.

NUTRITIONAL INFORMATION:
5 servings, 204 calories | 18.84 g fat 1.56 g of total carbohydrates 0.77 g of pure carbohydrates | 0.2 g of fibre 6.61 g of protein

❖ **Omelet Spanish Convey**

Preparation time: 10 minutes

Preparation time: 20 minutes

Total time: 30 minutes

Servings per package: 4

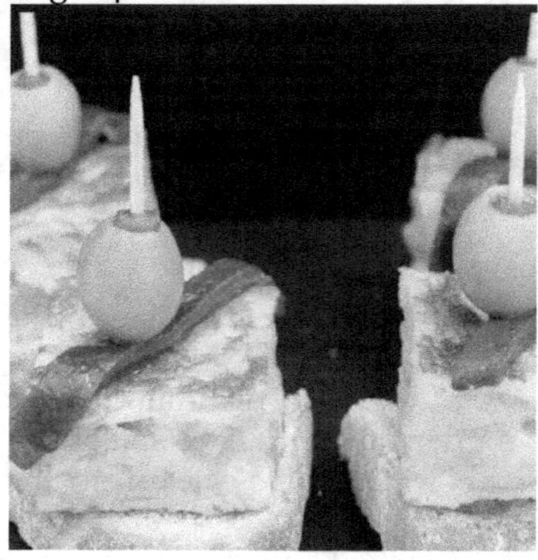

Ingredients:

- five eggs
- 1/4 cup chopped spinach
- 1/2 onion, diced
- two tablespoons coconut milk

- one teaspoon garlic, finely chopped
- four tablespoons avocado oil
- sea salt and freshly ground black pepper

Instructions:

1. Heat oil in a frying pan over medium heat. Add onions and garlic and fry for 1-2 minutes until soft.
2. Add spinach and cook another 4-5 minutes, remove from heat.
3. Break the eggs in a bowl, add coconut milk and season to taste. The beat is not yet well combined.
4. In another pan, heat the oil over medium heat, add half of the egg mixture into the pan and pour boiling until they are tough, to run.   Turn the tortilla over and place half of the spinach mixture on top, twist or fold the tortilla to coat the spinach.
5. Repeat this with the other half of the egg and spinach.
6. Cut the wraps in half and enjoy.

NUTRITIONAL INFORMATION:
4 servings, 227 calories | 21.04 g fat 2.4 g total carbohydrates 0.85 g of pure carbohydrates | 0.5 g of fibre 7.33 g of protein

❖ **Cashew Pancakes**

Preparation time: 5 minutes

Preparation time: 10 minutes

Total time: 15 minutes

Servings per package: 4

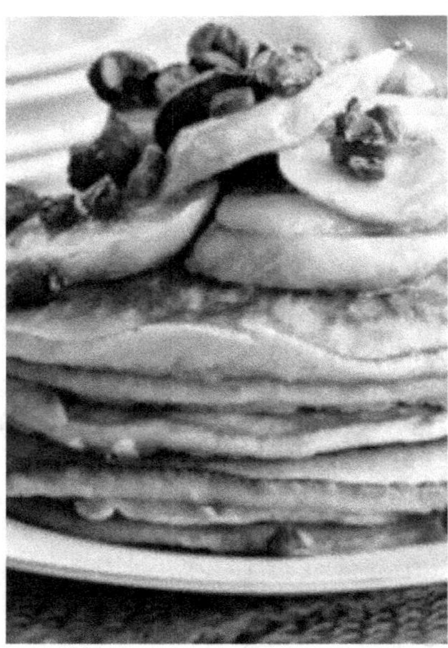

Ingredients:

- 2 grams of pork rind
- eight eggs
- eight tablespoons unsweetened cashew milk
- four teaspoons maple extract
- four teaspoons of ground cinnamon
- eight tablespoons coconut oil, for frying

Instructions:

1. Place the pig skins in a blender or food processor and press until finely powdered. (Alternatively, you can crush with a mortar or put it in a plastic bag and roll with a roller!)

2. Add the remaining ingredients (except coconut oil) and mix by hand until smooth.
3. Heat the pan over medium heat. After heating evenly, add one tablespoon of coconut oil.
4. Pour ¼ cup of dough into the pan.
5. Bake for about 2 minutes until the bottom is golden brown. Turn over and let the other side cook completely.

6. Remove the pancakes from the pan on the heating plate and place them in the oven (oven temperature is the lowest).
7. Repeat this with the remaining dough and add coconut oil to cook each pancake if necessary.
8. Remove the hot plate from the oven and serve hot pancakes!

NUTRITIONAL INFORMATION

44 grams of fat 1 g of total carbohydrates 1 g of pure carbohydrates 0 g of fibre 24 g of protein

❖ **Burrito Breakfast**

Preparation time: 5 minutes

Preparation time: 5 minutes

Total time: 10 minutes

Servings per package: 4

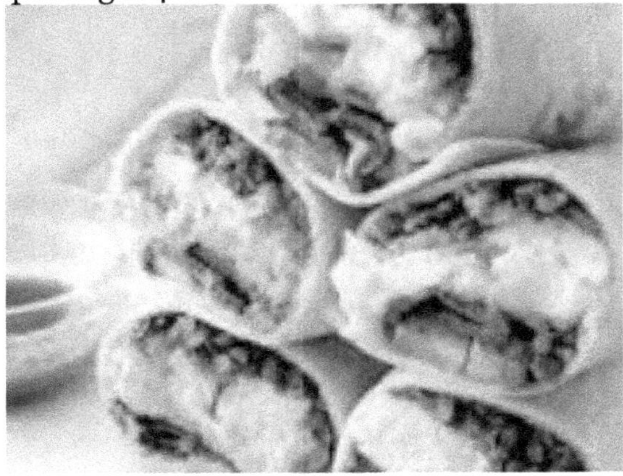

Ingredients:

FILLING:
- 4 oz breakfast sausage
- four eggs
- ½ cup of grated cheddar cheese
- ½ cup chopped soft spinach

- 1/3 cup diced onion
- 1/3 cup diced bell pepper
- a spoonful of olive oil

FOR ALMOND TORTILLA:
- 1.5 cups almond flour
- three tablespoons psyllium peeling powder
- 1/2 teaspoon baking powder
- 1/8 teaspoon of salt
- two proteins
- four tablespoons of boiling water
- 2 tablespoons deep-fry avocado oil

Instructions:

FOR TORTILLA:

1. Mix all tortilla ingredients in a small bowl; mix well.
2. Pour boiling water into the dough and mix with a spatula.
3. After all components have been mixed, allow the mixture to stand for 15 minutes.
4. Divide the dough into four equal parts.
5. Roll each portion into a ball and create a circle of 1/8 inch between two pieces of parchment paper.
6. Heat a large 10-inch pan over medium heat, and lightly coat the pan with avocado/olive oil.
7. Place the omelets in the pan and bake for 30 to 60 seconds on each side until golden brown. Turn and repeat on the other side.

8. Repeat with the remaining cakes.

FOR FILLING:

1. Heat half of the oil in a frying pan over medium heat.
2. Add onions and fry for a minute or two.
3. Add pepper and sausage, cook until the sausage is well cooked.
4. Remove fire and add spinach; Stir and let cool.
5. Divide the remaining oil into two pans. Put both on medium heat.

6. Put the beaten egg in the pan and stir to cover the entire pan. When the egg starts laying, turn it again to place the egg evenly around the pan.
7. When it is almost done, carefully turn the egg into the most giant pan and sprinkle it evenly with cheese on it.
8. Prepare only a minute and slide on the plate. This is your tortilla!
9. Place each of the four egg cookies on separate plates or together in a bowl.
10. Place a quarter of the sausage mixture on one side of each egg and a double tortilla.
11. Serve warm.

NUTRITIONAL INFORMATION:

Each Porting, 539.55 Calories | 44.39 g fat 14.05g Total Carbohydrates 6.18 g of pure carbohydrates | 7.87 g of fibre 25.22 g of protein

Chapter twelve: Lunch recipes

❖ Tikka of Mushrooms and Onion:

Preparation time: 30 minutes

Preparation time: 15 minutes

Total time: 45 minutes

Servings per package: 4

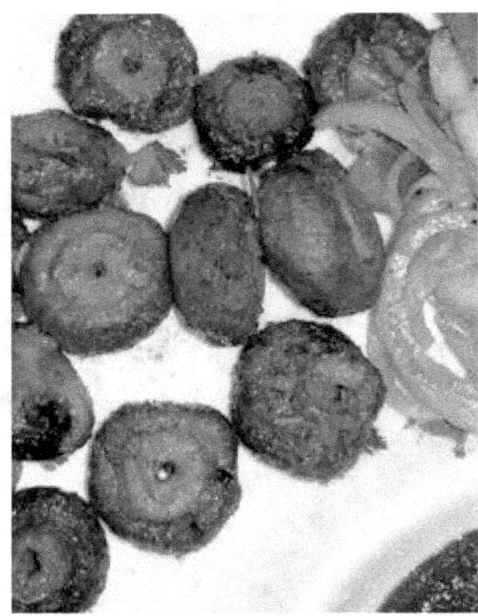

Ingredients:

- 2/3 cups thick whipped cream
- 1/3 teaspoon of cumin powder
- 2-1/2 tablespoons lemon juice
- 2-1/2 teaspoons of olive oil
- 3/4 teaspoon of ginger and garlic paste
- salt to taste
- 14 small mushrooms
- 2/3 onions, petals
- four teaspoons of olive oil, for baking
- wooden sticks

Instructions:

1. Take the first six ingredients in a large bowl, mix well to a make homogeneous mixture.
2. Add mushrooms and onions to this mixture and cover carefully. Cover and marinate in the fridge for 1 hour.
3. Preheat the oven to 425.
4. Put mushrooms and onions on wooden skewers.
5. Place in oven on a baking sheet or a baking tray for about 30 minutes, turning every 10 minutes to get a uniform preparation to guarantee.   Also grill the grill over medium heat and keep turning everywhere
6. Sprinkle with lemon juice to taste and serve immediately.

NUTRITIONAL INFORMATION:

4 servings, 153 calories 15.1 g fat 4.19 g total carbohydrates 1.23 g of pure carbohydrates 0.7 g of fiber 1.71 g of protein

❖ Feta Chick Spinach:

Total time: 10 minutes

Preparation time: 20 minutes

Total time: 30 minutes

Servings per package: 4 packages

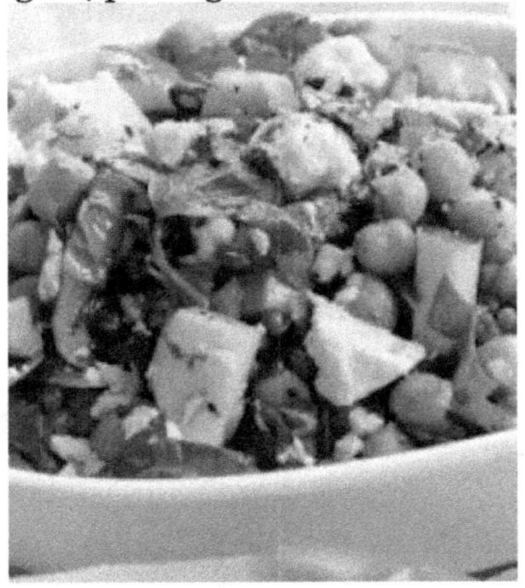

Ingredients:

FOR FILLING

- ½ cup of olives, cut into large pieces
- Four tablespoons grated feta cheese
- 1-1/2 tablespoons fresh lemon juice
- One tablespoon chopped fresh oregano
- 1/8 teaspoon ground black pepper
- 8 grams of boneless and boneless fried chicken fillet (about 1 cup)
- 12 spinach leaves

- 1 cup thick whipped cream

FOR ALMENDRAS OMELETS:
- 1.5 cups almond flour
- Three tablespoons psyllium peeling powder
- 1/2 teaspoon baking powder
- 1/8 teaspoon of salt
- Two proteins
- Four tablespoons of boiling water
- Two tablespoons avocado oil for frying

Instructions:

1. Mix all tortilla ingredients in a small bowl, mix well.
2. Pour boiling water into the dough and mix with a spatula.
3. Once all the ingredients have been mixed, let the dough stand for 15 minutes.
4. Divide the dough into four equal parts.
5. Roll each portion on a ball and make then a 1/8 inch thick circle between two pieces of parchment paper.
6. Heat a sizeable 10-inch pan over medium heat, lightly greased with avocado/olive oil.
7. Place the omelets in the pan and cook for 30 to 60 seconds on each side until golden brown. Turn and repeat on the other side.
8. Repeat this with the remaining cakes.
9. For the filling, mix all ingredients (except spinach and heavy cream) in a medium bowl and mix well.
10. Spread one tablespoon thick cream over each tortilla.
11. Divide the spinach into four pieces, place each portion on one edge of each tortilla.
12. Spoon ¼ of the mixture over the spinach filling and roll.

13. Repeat 3 more lozenges.
14. Halve and serve.

NUTRITIONAL INFORMATION

4 servings, 436 calories 31.54 g fat 6.65 g Total carbohydrates 1.53 g net Carbohydrates | 0.7 g of fiber 34.17 g of protein

❖ Asian Beef Salad:

Preparation time: 10 minutes

Preparation time: 20 minutes

Total time: 30 minutes

Servings per package: 5

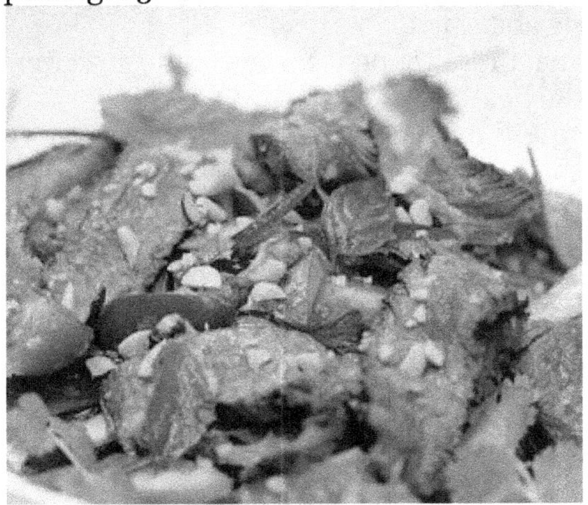

Ingredients:

- 24 grams of ground beef
- 1/2 tablespoon sesame oil
- ½ shredded onion
- ¼ cup tamari sauce
- two tablespoons of granular stevia
- one teaspoon chili and garlic sauce
- ½ teaspoon of garlic paste
- two teaspoons of chopped garlic
- ¼ cup chopped cashew nuts
- five green lettuce leaves
- salt and pepper to taste
- chives for decoration, minced

Instructions:

1. Heat ½ tablespoon sesame oil in a pan over medium heat.

2. Add the chopped onions to a hot pan, cook until smooth, and start baking.
3. Mix the minced meat and cook until the chicken is completely brown.
4. Add tamari sauce, stevia, chili and garlic sauce, ginger paste and chopped garlic.
5. Reduce the heat and cook the mixture until most of the liquid is absorbed.
6. Combine the chopped cashew nuts and remove the pan from the heat.
7. Allow the liquid to cool down for a few minutes and then add tablespoons of the meat mixture to the cups with the green lettuce.
8. Pour the chopped green onions before serving.

NUTRITIONAL INFORMATION:

each serving, 395 calories 31 grams of fat Total 4 g of carbohydrates 3.9 g of pure carbohydrates | 0.1 g of fiber 25 g of protein

❖ **Fried Pepper Soup:**

Preparation time 10 minutes

Preparation time 10 minutes

Total time: 20 minutes.

Servings per package: 4

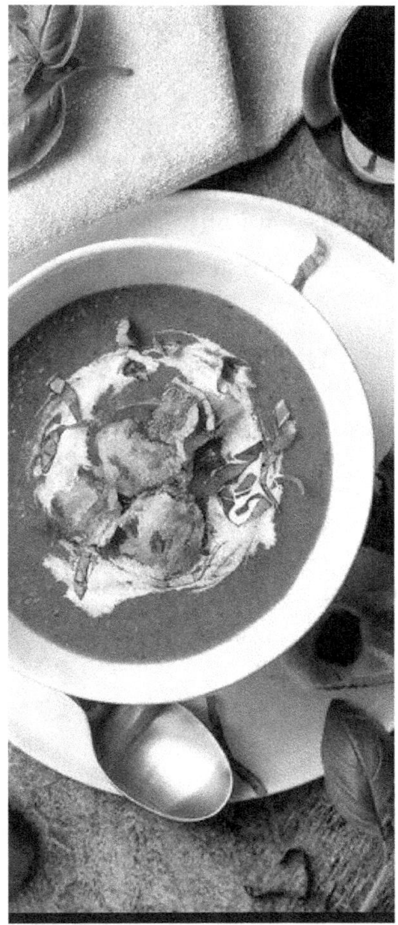

Ingredients:

- ¼ cup of olive oil
- 1 cup thick cream
- four teaspoons parmesan cheese
- four fried red peppers
- ¼ cup chopped onion
- one teaspoon garlic, finely chopped
- one teaspoon chili flakes
- ½ teaspoon of xanthan gum
- salt and pepper to taste

Instructions:

1. Mix red pepper in a blender until a thick sauce is formed.
2. Add onions, chili flakes, salt and pepper to a blender and grind again.
3. Heat the garlic in a pan and then add the red pepper mixture. Bring to boil. Mix the thick cream and boil again.
4. Combine xanthan gum and olive oil in a separate bowl.
5. Pour xanthan gum and olive oil into the soup.
6. Bring to the boil and pour the Parmesan cheese.
7. Serve hot.

NUTRITIONAL INFORMATION:
4 servings, 108 calories 2 grams of fat 17.3 g total carbohydrates 13.7 g of pure carbohydrates | 3.6 g of fiber 4.7 g of protein

❖ Avocado Chicken Salad:

Preparation time: 15 minutes

Preparation time: 10 minutes

Total time: 25 minutes

Servings per package: 4

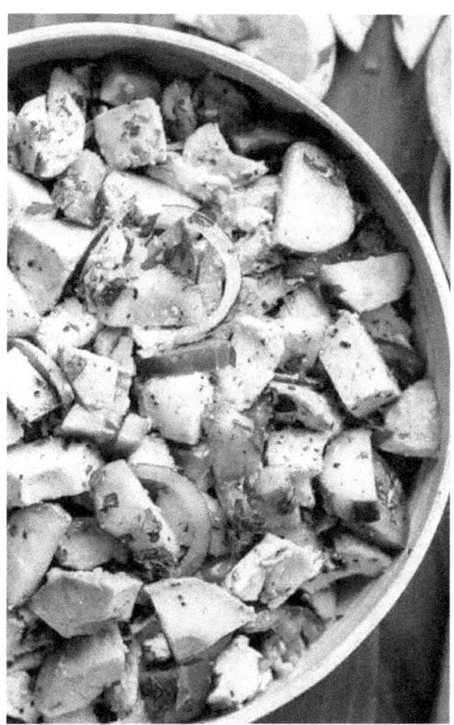

Ingredients:

- 2 avocados
- two chicken fillets (16 ounces)
- one chopped tomato
- ½ shredded onion
- one celery stalk, finely chopped
- two tablespoons mayonnaise
- one tablespoon lemon juice
- one tablespoon of olive oil
- salt and pepper to taste.

Instructions:

1. Cut the chicken into smaller pieces than the slice and season with salt and pepper on the sides.
2. Cut each avocado in half and remove the seeds. Remove the avocado pulp with a spoon and store.
3. Add olive oil to the pan over medium heat. Add chicken to the pan and cook well. Let cool.

4. While the chicken cools, chop the tomatoes, onions and celery and place them in a bowl.
5. Grind the avocado meat in a separate bowl so that it is relatively smooth, add it to the mixing bowl.
6. Add mayonnaise and cooled chicken and mix all ingredients well.
7. Pour a small scoop of the avocado peel with a mixture of avocado, chicken and vegetables.
8. Sprinkle each with lemon juice and season with salt and pepper.

NUTRITIONAL INFORMATION:
Each portion, 360 calories 29.5 g of fat 8.6 g total carbohydrates 3 g of pure carbohydrates 3.6 g of fiber 17 g of protein

Chapter thirteen: Dinner Recipes

❖ **Mushroom Meat Creamy:**

Preparation time: 5 minutes

Preparation time: 25 minutes.

Total time: 30 minutes

Servings per package: 4

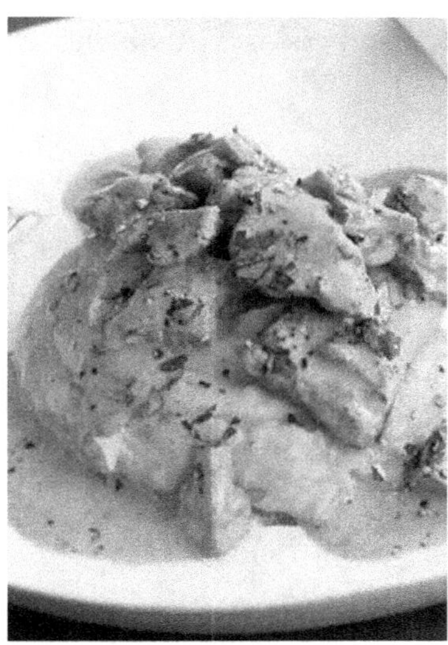

Ingredients:

- 4 tenderloin
- Three tablespoons peanut butter
- One tablespoon olive oil
- One teaspoon garlic, finely chopped
- 1 pound of milk thistle
- Salt and ground pepper to taste
- 1/4 cup low-sodium chicken broth
- 1/2 cup thick cream
- chopped fresh parsley to decorate

Instructions:

1. Heat a 10-inch cast-iron skillet over medium heat, add olive oil.
2. Once the olive oil is hot, add the tenderloin and cook for 10-15 minutes until done, if desired.
3. Place the meat on a plate and reserve.
4. Add peanut butter in the same pan used for meat.
5. Once the peanut butter has melted, add the garlic and leave it on the fire for 2 minutes.
6. Add mushrooms, cook for 3-4 minutes over medium heat.
7. Season with salt and pepper and mix well.
8. Add chicken broth and whipped cream and cook for 4-5 minutes.

9. Pour the sauce and cooked mushrooms over the meat.
10. Serve hot.

NUTRITIONAL INFORMATION:

One serving of 388 calories | 24.67 g fat | Total 9.8 g carbohydrates | 3.87 g of pure carbohydrates 3.3 g of fibre 33.38 g of protein

❖ Lambar Chops:

Preparation time: 5 minutes

Preparation time: 20 minutes

Total time: 25 minutes

Servings per package: 4

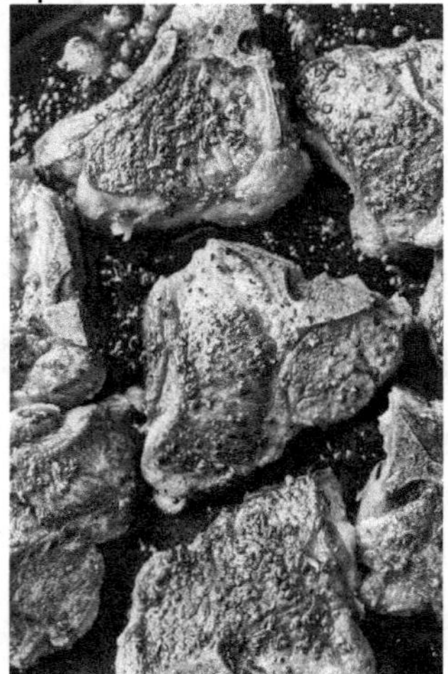

Ingredients:

- 4 lamb chops
- one tablespoon olive oil
- salt and pepper to taste
- 4 oz. butter
- ¼ cup chopped parsley
- one lemon, in segments

Instructions:

1. Heat the pan over medium heat, add oil and butter.
2. Once the butter and butter are warm, add the lamb chops and fry them for about 8-10 minutes.
3. As soon as the lamb chops are cooked, they get a pleasant brown color, and the liquid disappears.
4. Sprinkle with chopped parsley.
5. Serve hot.

NUTRITIONAL INFORMATION:

one portion, 301 calories 29.34 g fat 2.15 g total carbohydrates 0.92 g of pure carbohydrates | 0.3 g of fibers | 9.01 g of protein

❖ **Brazilian Fish:**

Preparation time: 15 minutes

Preparation time: 40 minutes

Total time: 55 minutes

Servings per package: 5

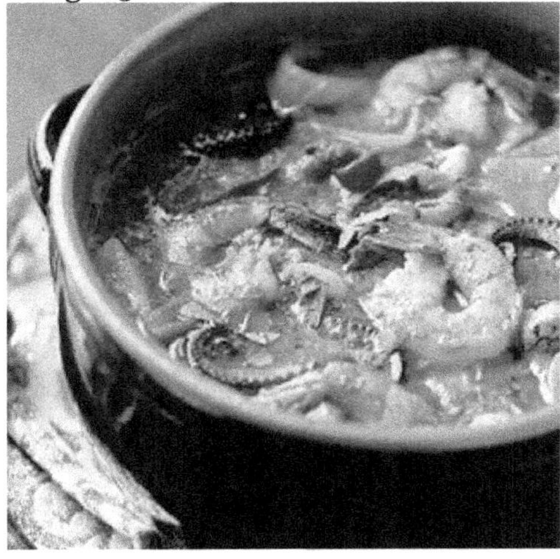

Ingredients:

FOR BASE OF STEW:

- one onion, diced
- one chopped red pepper
- five cloves of chopped garlic
- one can of 14 ounce chopped tomatoes.
- 8 grams of fish or vegetable broth
- 6 grams of canned coconut milk, full of fat
- two tablespoons coconut oil
- one tablespoon ground cumin
- one tablespoon bell pepper
- one tablespoon of olive oil
- one teaspoon of salt
- ½ teaspoon of black pepper
- ¼ to ½ teaspoon of cayenne pepper (to taste)

FOR FINISH:

- 24 grams of solid white fish (cod / halibut, etc.)
- Two tablespoons coconut oil
- One tablespoon lime juice
- One tablespoon coriander or chopped fresh parsley

Instructions:

1. Combine lime juice, olive oil, salt and pepper in a large bowl. Add the fish and mix until well covered.
2. Set aside.
3. Heat the oil in a large frying pan over medium heat. Add garlic, onion and pepper and fry until they are soft, about 2 to 3 minutes.
4. Pour in stock and coconut milk, mix well. Add caraway, pepper and pepper, keep stirring.
5. Bring the soup to the boil, simmer and add the fish.
6. Cover and cook until the fish is separated about 12-15 minutes.
7. Serve with fresh parsley/coriander as a side dish and enjoy!

NUTRITIONAL INFORMATION:

Each portion, 320 calories 18 grams of fat Total 10 g of carbohydrates 7 g of pure carbohydrates 3 g of fibre 27 g of protein

❖ **Big Hamburger:**

Preparation time: 6 minutes

Preparation time: 12 min.

Total time: 18 minutes.

Servings per package: 4

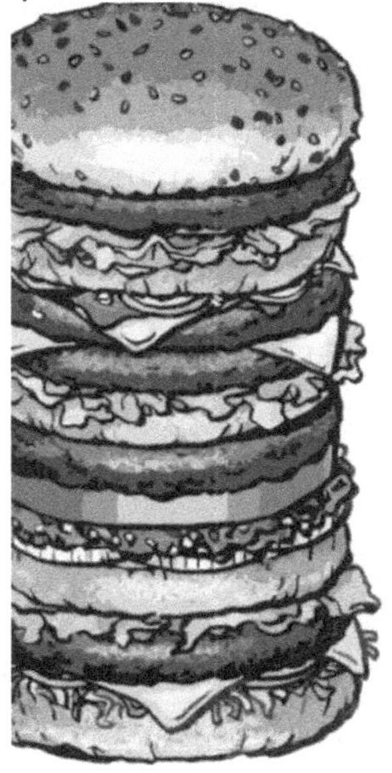

Ingredients:

FOR CIVIL:

- two tablespoons of green chili paste
- 2 pounds of ground beef
- two chicken stock cubes
- 4 grams of cheddar cheese

FOR AMK:

- ¾ cup of almond flour
- Two teaspoons of baking powder
- Six tablespoons of olive oil
- Four eggs

Instructions:

Sandwich:

1. Add baking powder and almond flour in a medium bowl. Mix well.
2. Add butter and egg.
3. Beat all ingredients with a fork
4. Divide the mixture evenly into four bowls. (Pending: use a bowl with a bottom the size you want for sandwiches to be)

5. Microwave, a head (AMK) in a ship in up to 90 seconds.

6. Cut the centre of the bun with a bread knife to make the top and bottom of the bun.
7. Optional: toasted or toasted bread

Hamburger:

1. Heat the grill on high heat.
2. Combine the meat and diced green chili peppers in a medium bowl.
3. Crush a piece of stock powder and work with minced meat.

4. Form 4 empanadas.
5. Lightly grease the grid and bake the patties for 5 minutes on each side or until you prefer.
6. Cover each cake with cheese in about 2 minutes before removing it from the grill.
7. Serve in sandwiches and enjoy!

NUTRITIONAL INFORMATION:
each serving, 1087 calories 92.67 g fat 13.7 g total carbohydrates 8.75 g of pure carbohydrates 4.95 g of fiber 56 g of protein

❖ **Big Hamburger:**

Preparation time: 6 minutes

Preparation time: 12 min.

Total time: 18 minutes.

Dosages per package: 4

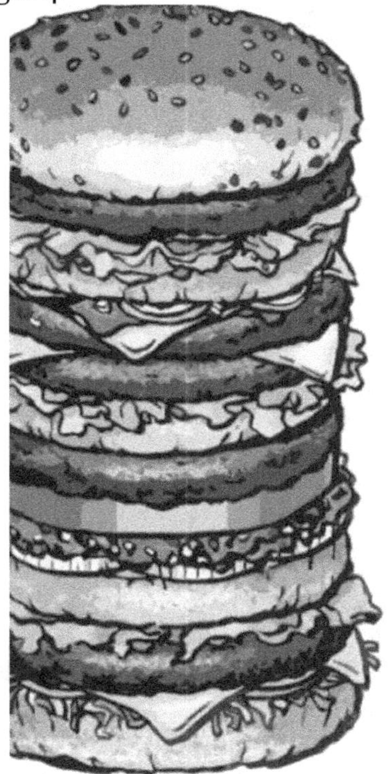

Ingredients:

FOR HAMBURGER:

- Two tablespoons green chili paste

- 2 pounds ground beef
- Two cubes of chicken broth
- 4 oz cheddar cheese

FOR BALL:

- ¾ cup of almond flour
- Two teaspoons baking powder
- Six tablespoons olive oil
- Four eggs

Instructions:

Sandwich:

1. Add baking powder and almond flour in a medium bowl. Mix well
2. Add butter and egg.
3. Beat all ingredients well with a fork
4. Divide the mixture evenly into four bowls. (Pending: use a bowl with a bottom from which you want the sandwiches)

5. Microwave one bowl (lunch) at a time, for 90 seconds at high temperature.
6. Cut the middle part of the bun with a bread knife to make the top and bottom of the bun.
7. Optional: toasted or toasted bread

Hamburger:

1. Preheat the grill on high heat.
2. Combine the meat and the diced green chili peppers in a medium bowl.
3. Crush the bouillon cube until it becomes powder and work with the meat.
4. Form 4 empanadas.
5. Lightly grease the grill and grilled patties for 5 minutes per side, or until you prefer.
6. Cover each cake with cheese about 2 minutes before you remove it from the grill.
7. Serve in sandwiches and enjoy!

NUTRITIONAL INFORMATION:

each serving, 1087 calories 92.67 g fat 13.7 g total carbohydrates 8.75 g of pure carbohydrates 4.95 g of fiber 56 g of protein

❖ South Fried Chicken:

Preparation time: 35 minutes

Preparation time: 10 minutes

Total time: 45 minutes

Dosages per package: 6

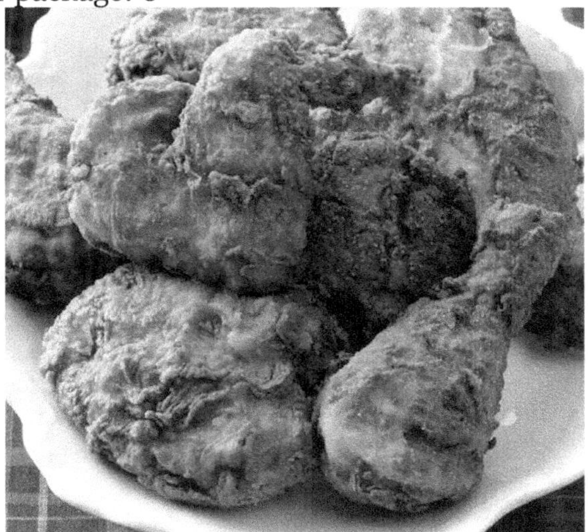

INGREDIENTS:

- 2 pounds Chicken pieces
- one egg
- ½ cup almond flour
- one teaspoon garlic powder
- ½ teaspoon of chili powder
- two teaspoons of celery salt
- one teaspoon of oregano
- two tablespoons of thick cream
- ½ cup of grated Parmesan cheese

Instructions:

1. Preheat the fryer to 180 degrees.
2. Combine celery salt, garlic powder, chili powder and oregano in a large bowl.
3. Put the chicken in the bowl and mix well. Leave in the fridge for 30 minutes.
4. Beat eggs and cream together. In another bowl, combine almond flour and grated Parmesan cheese.
5. Dip each piece of chicken in the egg mixture and then roll the almond/parmesan flour mixture.
6. Once the whole chicken is covered, place it in a frying basket and cook for about 8 minutes until it is golden brown.
7. Sprinkle with parsley and serve.

NUTRITIONAL INFORMATION:

Each serving, 214 calories each | 8 grams of fat 0.07 g total carbohydrates 0.06 g of pure carbohydrates | 0.1 g of fiber 34 g of protein

❖ Rancho Del Rey Chicken Soup:

Preparation time: 5 minutes

Preparation time: 20 minutes

Total time: 25 minutes

Servings per package: 6

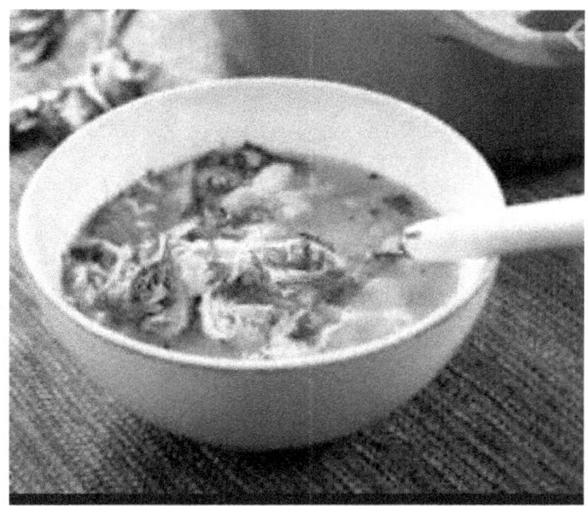

Ingredients:

- Eight tablespoons of oil
- ½ cup of heavy cream
- 2 cups of Mexican cheese mix
- Fresh coriander, chopped (to taste)
- 2.5 pounds of chicken fillet
- 4 cups of chicken broth
- 10 - gram can of diced tomatoes w / green chili peppers

- one jalapeno cut into cubes.
- ¼ cup coconut flour
- four teaspoons of chili powder
- one tablespoon ground cumin
- one tablespoon garlic powder
- 1 ½ teaspoon of xanthan gum
- one teaspoon of salt
- pepper to taste

Instructions:

1. Melt the butter in a pan over medium heat and mix in the coconut flour. Mix well.
2. Combine chicken broth, chili powder, garlic powder, cumin, pepper and salt.
3. Add chicken, tomatoes with green chili and jalapenos.

4. Cover the pan and cook for 15 minutes. Release the heat when you're done. Mix xanthan gum, cheese and whipped cream.
5. Serve hot.

NUTRITIONAL INFORMATION:

Each Serving, 329 Calories Each | 20.6 g fat Total 2 g of carbohydrates 2 g of pure carbohydrates 0 g of fibre 32 g of protein

❖ Chile White Chicken:

Preparation time: 5 minutes

Preparation time: 40 minutes

Total time: 45 minutes

Servings per package: 6

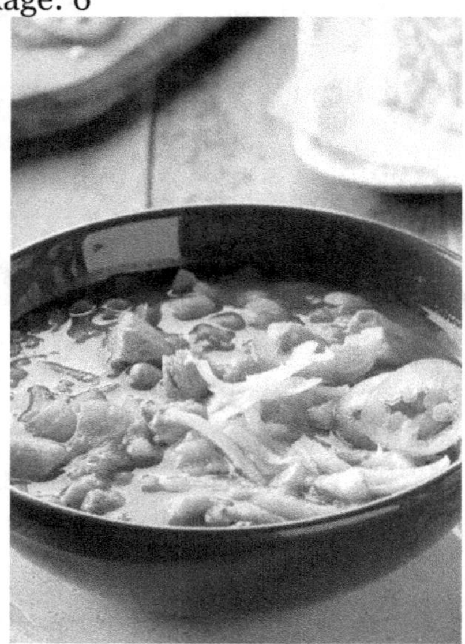

INGREDIENTS:

- Two tablespoons butter
- 1 cup thick cream

- 2 cups of sour cream
- 4 cups of chicken broth
- Ten chicken thighs (with skin), cut into cubes
- 1 pound of chopped cauliflower
- One onion, diced
- 14 grams diced green chili
- Two teaspoons of oregano
- Two teaspoons of cumin
- Two teaspoons of salt
- One teaspoon pepper

Instructions:

1. In a saucepan over medium heat, add butter, onions and chicken and cook until the chicken is ready.
2. Add chili, caraway, oregano, salt, pepper and cauliflower. Mix well.
3. Add chicken stock, stir and cover the pan.
4. Cook for 30 minutes on high heat.
5. Let off steam and open the pan.
6. Add thick cream and sour cream, hot to high.
7. Serve

NUTRITIONAL INFORMATION:

Each serving, 843 calories each | 64.18 g fat | 10.56 g total carbohydrates 7.68 g of pure carbohydrates | 2.88 g of fibre 58.7 g of protein

❖ **Crusty Broccoli:**

Preparation time: 15 minutes

Preparation time: 40 minutes

Total time: 55 minutes

Servings per package: 6

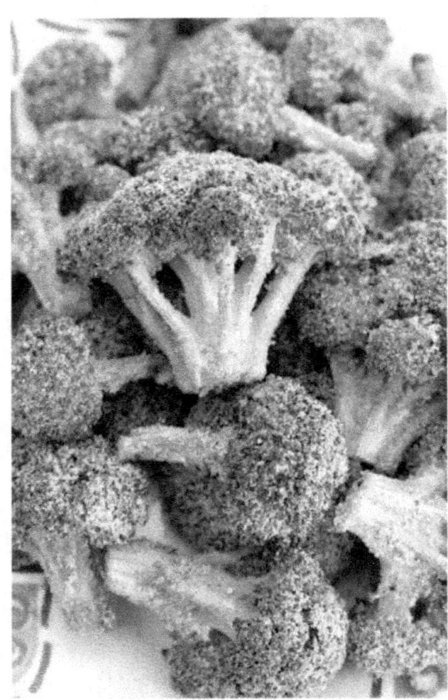

Ingredients:

- 3 cups of chopped broccoli florets
- 1 cup of grated cheddar cheese
- 1 cup of coconut milk
- ½ cup of coconut cream
- Five large eggs
- ¾ teaspoon of sea salt
- 1/8 teaspoon ground black pepper
- One tablespoon grease olive oil

Instructions:

1. Preheat the oven to 350°.
2. Cook chopped broccoli until soft, crispy and bright green.
3. Grease the baking dish with olive oil and put the broccoli in a greased form.
4. Combine milk, cream, eggs, salt and black pepper in a bowl.
5. Pour the mixture on a plate, cover with grated cheddar cheese.

6. Bake in a preheated oven for 35-40 minutes until the middle is done.
7. Cut the cake into six pieces and serve.

NUTRITIONAL INFORMATION:
Each serving 339 calories | 30.72 g fat | Total 4.84 g of carbohydrates 1.24 g of pure carbohydrates | 1.9 g of fiber 13.45 g of protein

Chapter fourteen: Seafood recipe

❖ **Cajun tuna remoulade**

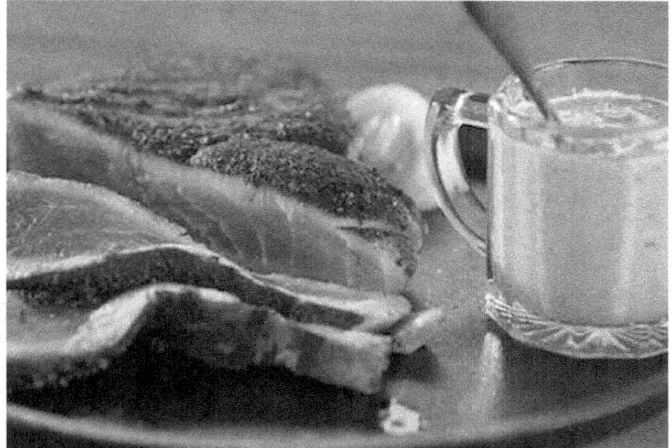

❖
Ingredients:

- ¼ cups of real mayonnaise
- A pinch of pepper
- One tablespoon chopped dill
- One teaspoon fresh lemon juice, freshly squeezed
- ½ teaspoon of Dijon mustard
- one skewer organic cucumber
- ½ tsp spice mixes
- Two large hard-boiled eggs, chopped
- 12 ounces of tuna without bone, sliced
- One tablespoon olive oil

Instructions:

1. Mix all ingredients except eggs and tuna in a bowl. Place the remolded on the side.
2. Heat the olive oil in a frying pan over medium heat, lay the steak and season with salt and pepper. Cook on each side for 3 minutes.

3. Serve tuna with chopped eggs and remolded.

NUTRITIONAL INFORMATION:
Calories per serving: 528; Carbohydrates: 2.1 g; Protein: 46.1 g; Fat: 35.7 g; Fiber: 0.3 g

❖ **Fried Asian Salmon With Bok Choy:**

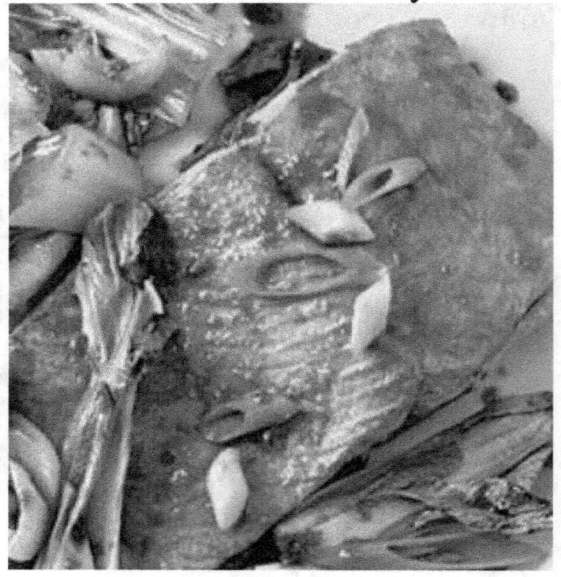

Ingredients:

- juice of 1 lemon, freshly squeezed
- Two tablespoons biological tamari
- 12 grams sliced salmon boneless
- pinch of salt and pepper
- ½ tablespoon oil
- 2/3 tablespoons of olive oil
- 6 ounces of mushrooms, sliced

Instructions:

1. Preheat the oven to 475 F.
2. Mix lemon juice and tamari in a bowl. Set aside.
3. Season the salmon with salt and pepper. Put in a bowl and pour ½ mixture of tamari sauce. Let marinate in the fridge for 15 minutes.
4. While the salmon is marinating, heat your oil in a saucepan over medium heat. Pour onto a baking sheet after melting.

5. Place the chopped salmon on a baking sheet and place it in the oven for 10 minutes.
6. Meanwhile, heat the olive oil in a pan and fry the cabbage and mushrooms slices.
7. Serve salmon with baked vegetables.

NUTRITIONAL INFORMATION:
Calories per serving: 487; Carbohydrates: 10.1 g; Protein: 5 g; Fat: 25.8 g; Fiber : 7.3 g

❖ **Asian lobster salad:**

Ingredients:

- ¾ pound lobster, chopped
- 2 cups chopped Chinese cabbage
- ½ red bell pepper, chopped
- Four green onions, finely chopped
- One tablespoon roasted sesame seeds
- Two tablespoons unsweetened rice vinegar
- Two tablespoons of sauce tamari
- one teaspoon grated ginger
- One tablespoon vegetable oil
- One teaspoon of sesame oil

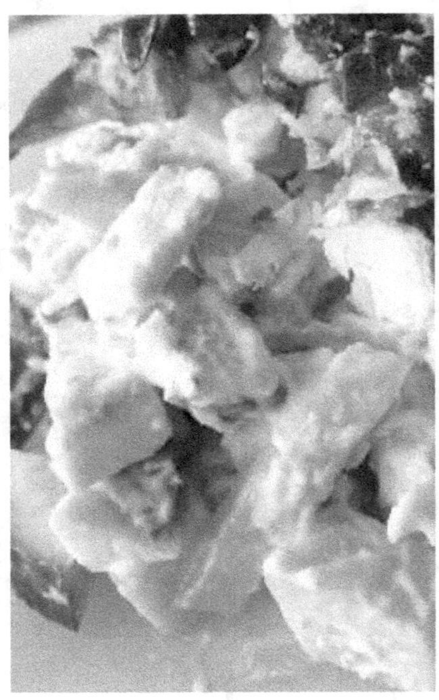

Instructions:

1. Combine lobster meat, cabbage, pepper and green onions in a bowl. Mix sesame seeds and mix.
2. Mix the remaining ingredient in another bowl. It becomes a salad dressing.
3. Pour salad dressing.

NUTRITIONAL INFORMATION:
Calories per serving: 325; Carbohydrates: 4.2 g; Protein: 38.9 g; Fat: 14 g; Fiber: 3 g

❖ **Halibut Bahiano:**

For four persons

Ingredients:

*   Two tablespoons olive oil

- Two tablespoons of freshly squeezed lemon juice
- 2-pound halibut fillet
- One teaspoon of chopped garlic
- Four tablespoons chopped onion
- 1 cup chopped green pepper
- One serrano, chopped
- One teaspoon salt
- ½ cup coconut cream
- One whole red tomato, chopped

Instructions:

1. In a small bowl, mix one tablespoon of olive oil and lemon juice.
2. Pour on halibut fillet and make sure the fish is covered with marinade.
3. Heat the remaining olive oil in a frying pan over medium-high heat. Fry onion and garlic until fragrant. Add bell pepper and Serrano bell pepper.
4. Place the fish slices on top and sprinkle with salt.
5. Add coconut cream and tomatoes.
6. Cover the pan and let it boil.
7. Reduce heat and allow 9 minutes simmer.

NUTRITIONAL INFORMATION:
Calories per serving: 400; Carbohydrates: 3.2 g; Protein: 48.6 g; Fat: 19.5 g; Fiber: 1.8 g

❖ **Smoked fish with broccoli:**

Portions: 1

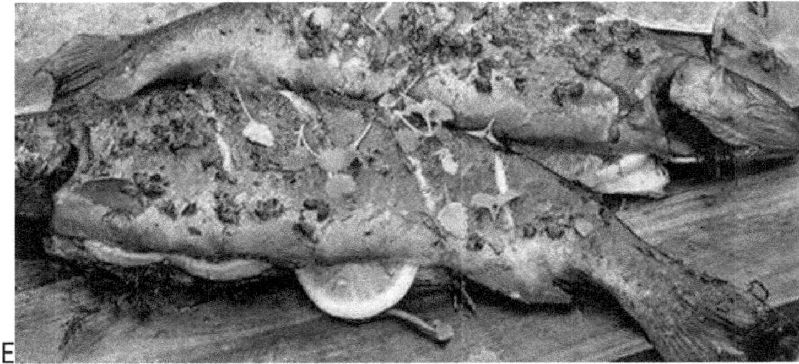

Ingredients:

- 6 grams of wild catfish
- Salt and pepper to taste.
- 1 cup chopped broccoli florets
- One tablespoon butter
- One tablespoon Italian spice mix

Instructions:

1. Preheat the oven to 350 F.
2. Place the catfish on a baking sheet covered with foil.
3. Season the fish with salt and pepper.
4. Arrange broccoli florets around the fish and sprinkle with an Italian spice mixture.
5. Put the oil on the fish.
6. Fold the side edges of the sheet to make a sealed package.
7. Put the fish in the oven and bake for 15 minutes.

NUTRITIONAL INFORMATION:
Calories per serving: 362; Carbohydrates: 4.5 g; Protein: 28.7 g; Fat: 25.9 g; Fiber: 2.2 g

❖ **Baked salmon with vegetables:**

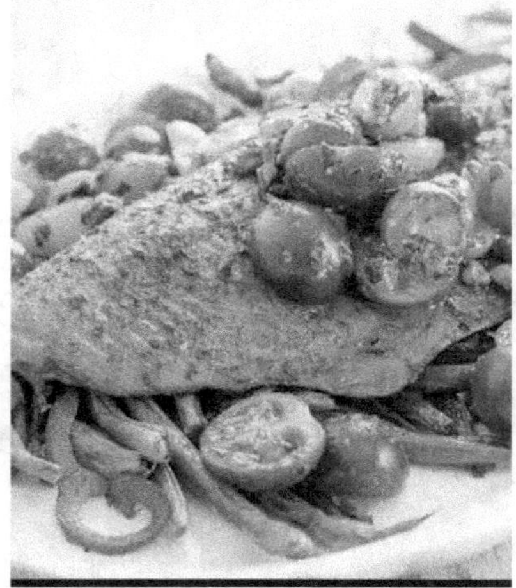

❖

Ingredients:

- ½ tablespoon olive oil
- ¼ tablespoon of butter
- 6 grams of wild Atlantic salmon
- Salt and pepper to taste.
- ¾ cup of chopped pears
- 8 grams of Chinese cabbage
- 2 grams of pickled okra
- 3 grams of red pepper, sown and sliced
- 1 cup diced tomatoes
- One tablespoon of vinegar sherry

Instructions:

1. Preheat the oven to 475 F.
2. Heat the oil and butter in a large cast-iron frying pan over medium heat until the butter has melted.
3. Season the fish to taste with salt and pepper to taste and place the meat face down in the pan.
4. Place the pan in the oven and bake for 10 minutes while turning the fish over at half the cooking time.
5. Add peas, cabbage and okra.
6. Put in the oven and cook for another 30 minutes or until the vegetables are dry.
7. Meanwhile, mix red pepper, tomatoes and sherry vinegar in a food processor. Season with salt and pepper.
8. Serve with mashed salmon and vegetables.

NUTRITIONAL VALUE:
calories per serving: 623; Carbohydrates: 7.9 g; Protein: 37.5 g; Fat: 44.1 g; Fiber: 2.3 g

❖ **Steamed lobster with butter:**

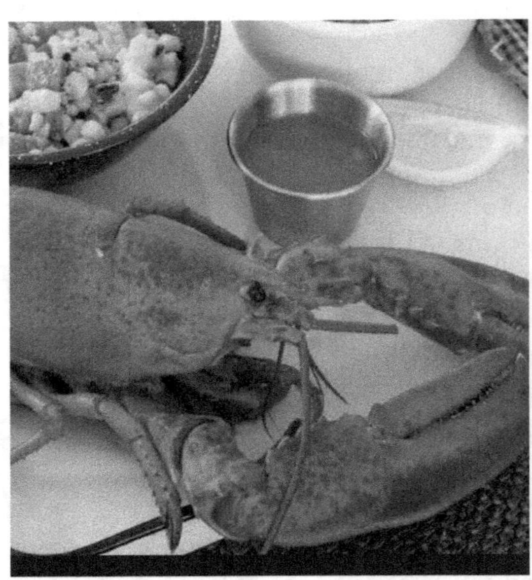

For four persons

Ingredients:

- Four lobsters
- ¾ cup unsalted butter
- ½ lemon, sliced

Instructions:

1. Boil 10 liters of water. Add salt.
2. Place the lobsters in a pan of boiling water and ensure that they are completely covered. Cook for 20 minutes.
3. Remove the lobsters from boiling water and place them on a paper towel.
4. Serve with butter and lemon slices.

NUTRITIONAL INFORMATION:
calories per serving: 442; Carbohydrates: 0.3 g; Protein: 28.6 g; Fat: 35.9 g; Fiber: 0 g

❖ **Blackened salmon:**

Servings: 2

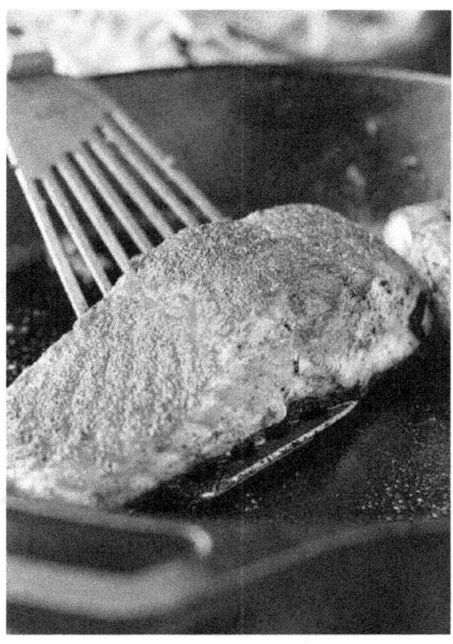

Ingredients:

- Three teaspoons of thyme, dried
- Three teaspoons of oregano dried leaves
- One tablespoon of spices old
- Salt and pepper to taste.
- ¼ cup of vegetable oil
- 24 ounces salmon boning

Instructions:

1. Mix thyme, oregano and old bay leaves in a bowl. Add salt and pepper.
2. Use two tablespoons of oil and cover the fish so that the herbs stick easily to the salmon meat.
3. Heat the remaining oil in a pan over medium heat.
4. Add fish and brown until the herb layer turns black. Do all sides for at least 3 minutes.

NUTRITIONAL INFORMATION:
calories per serving: 483; Carbohydrates: 0.7 g; Protein: 34.9 g; Fat: 36.8 g; Fiber: 0 g

❖ **Lobster grilled with garlic butter:**

Servings: 3

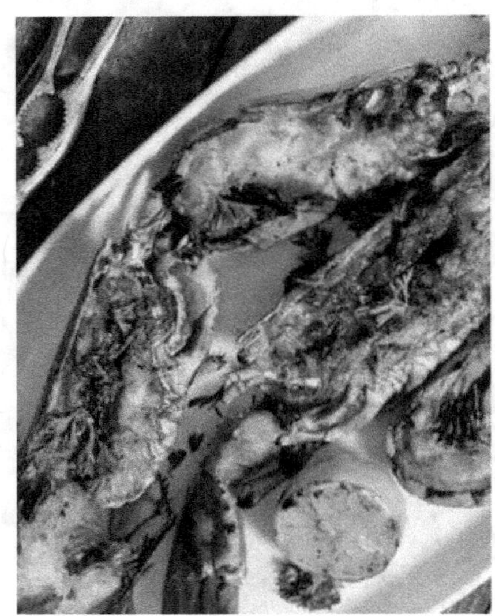

Ingredients:

- one teaspoon of garlic
- ¼ extra cups - olive oil
- One tablespoon melted butter
- 3 pounds of lobster
- 1/8 teaspoon salt

Instructions:

1. Preheat the oven to 350 F.
2. Mix the garlic, olive oil and oil in a bowl.
3. Divide the lobster into yourself.
4. Spread the lobster with a mixture of garlic and oil.
5. Season with salt.
6. Put in the oven and bake for 7 minutes.

NUTRITIONAL VALUE:
calories per serving: 303; Carbohydrates: 0 g; Protein: 42.7 g; Fat: 13.3 g; Fiber: 0 g

❖ **Custard Glaze Salmon:**

Servings: 4

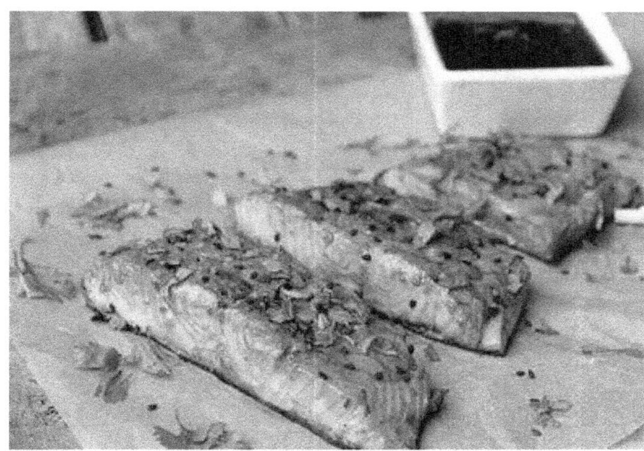

Ingredients:

- ¼ cup maple syrup
- ½ cup tap water
- Three teaspoons of Dijon mustard
- Two cloves, finely chopped
- ¼ teaspoon salt
- 2 pounds of wild Atlantic salmon

Instructions:

1. Mix all ingredients except salmon in a pan.
2. Let it brew until the sauce is reduced by approximately half. Allow cooling completely.
3. Preheat the grill and lay the skin of the salmon fillet.
4. Cook for 6 minutes on each side.
5. While cooking, pour salmon with sauce.

NUTRITIONAL INFORMATION:
calories per serving: 485; Carbohydrates: 0 g; Protein: 46.4 g; Fat: 30.4 g; Fiber: 0 g

❖ **Leftover tuna and artichoke salad:**

Servings: 3

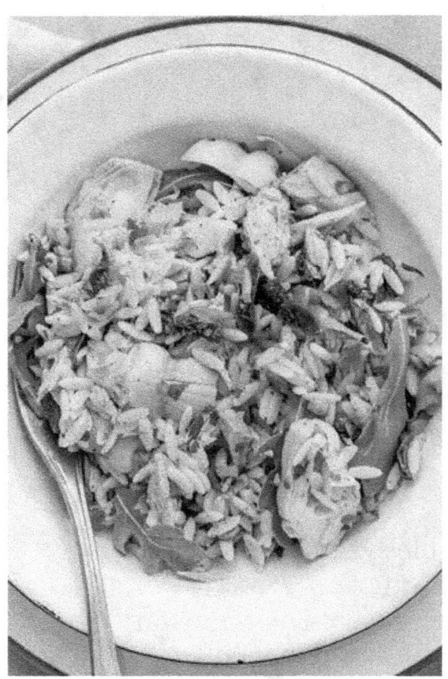

Ingredients:

- 4 grams of surplus tuna
- Six pieces of pickled artichokes, minced
- Two tablespoons egg mayonnaise
- 2 cups of Roman lettuce
- Salt and pepper to taste.

Instructions:

1. Combine all ingredients in a bowl.
2. Mix gently to coat all ingredients.
3. Adjust the herbs.

NUTRITIONAL INFORMATION:

Calories per serving: 464; Carbohydrates: 3.5 g; Protein: 3 2.7 g; Fat: 33.7 g; Fiber: 1.2 g

❖ **Salad with Tuna And Celery In Baby Spinach:**

Servings: 4

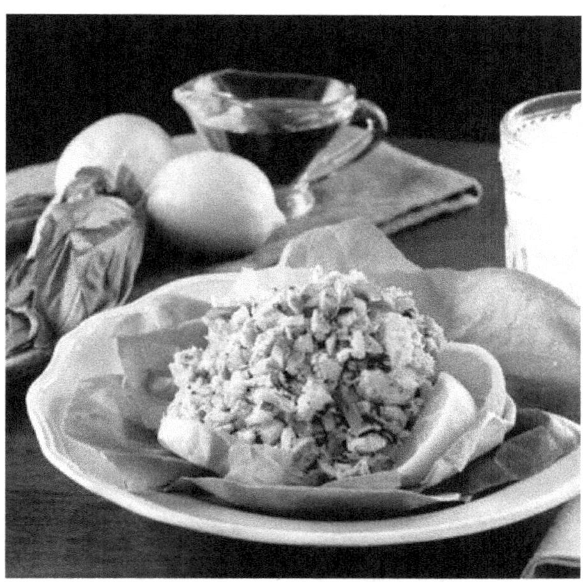

Ingredients:

- 5 grams of tuna packed in water, low in sodium
- One medium-sized chopped celery
- Two tablespoons of real egg mayonnaise
- 1 ½ cup spinach, rinse and grated
- Salt and pepper to taste.

Instructions:

1. Combine all ingredients in a bowl.
2. Mix gently to cover the ingredients with mayonnaise.
3. Cool before use in the refrigerator.

NUTYRITIONAL INFORMATION:
Calories per serving: 483; Carbohydrates: 2 g; Protein: 3 8.6 g; Fat: 33.5 g; Fiber: 1.3 g

❖ **Chilean Sea Bass with Ginger Broth:**

Servings: 2

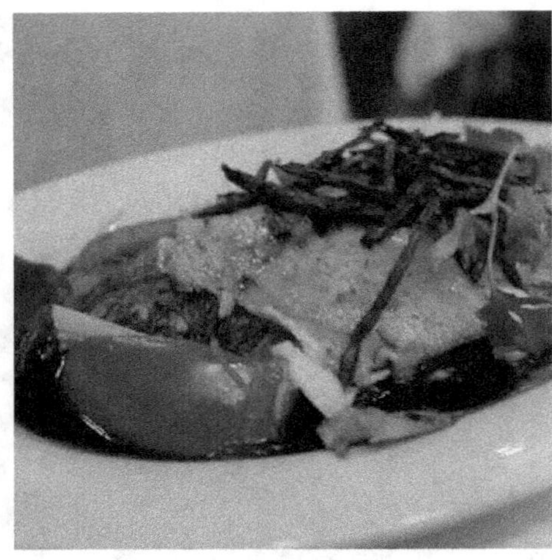

Ingredients:

- Two tablespoons olive oil
- 5 ½ tablespoons grated ginger
- 3 cups of sodium broth with low sodium
- One red pepper diced
- One chopped onion
- 1 tablespoon tomato paste
- ¼ teaspoon salt
- ½ cup cilantro, for decoration

Instructions:

1. Heat olive oil in a pan over medium heat.
2. Add ginger and stir for 3 minutes until light brown. Use a spoon with a slot and transfer ginger to a bowl. Set aside.
3. Pour the chicken stock into the same pan and place the pepper, fish, onion and tomato puree.
4. Season with salt.
5. Cook for 3 minutes and then cook for another 5 minutes.
6. Serve the coriander soup and pour the baked ginger.

NUTRITIONAL INFORMATION:

Calories per serving: 278; Carbohydrates: 0.7 g; Protein: 42.7 g; Fat: 9.4 g; Fiber: 0 g

❖ **Citrus Chili Shrimp:**

Servings: 2

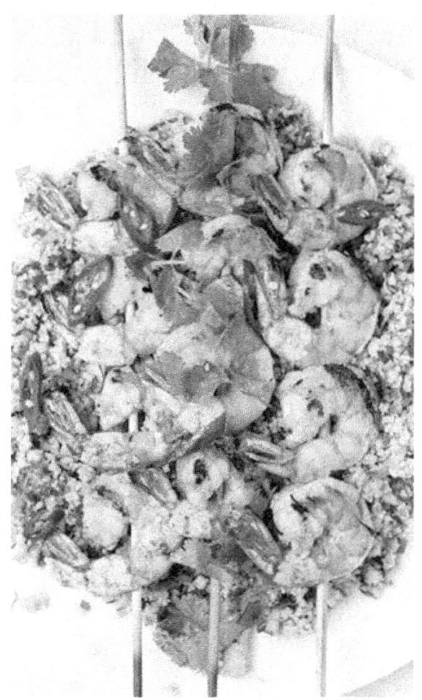

Ingredients:

- Seven tablespoons of olive oil
- 1/3 cup of freshly squeezed orange juice
- Two tablespoons grated orange peel
- ½ tablespoon freshly squeezed lime juice
- ¼ teaspoon of red pepper flakes
- ¼ teaspoon of cumin
- 1 ½ pounds shrimp, dish and deveined
- ½ teaspoon salt
- One tablespoon unsalted butter

Instructions:

1. In a bowl, mix six tablespoons of olive oil, orange juice, orange zest, lime juice, red pepper flakes, and caraway seeds. Add shrimp and season with salt. Let marinate for at least 30 minutes.

2. Melt the butter in a pan over medium heat and heat the remaining one tablespoon of olive oil.
3. Add pickled shrimp, including marinade.
4. Stir constantly for 3 minutes or until the shrimp turn pink.

NUTRITIONAL INFORMATION:
Calories per serving: 285; Carbohydrates: 1.2 g; Protein: 23.2 g; Fat: 20.3 g; Fiber: 0.1 g

❖ **Salmon Fillet with Citrus and Chili:**

Servings: 2

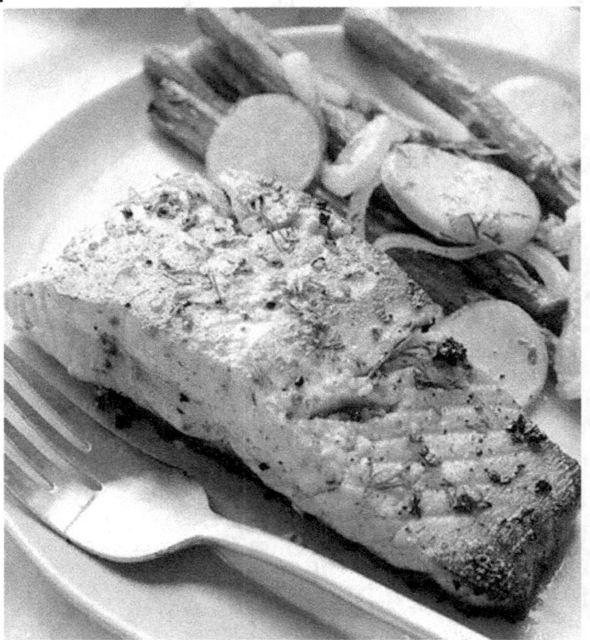

Ingredients:

- One teaspoon grated lemon zest
- One teaspoon grated orange peel
- Two tablespoons of freshly squeezed lemon juice
- One tablespoon olive oil
- Two tablespoons chili powder
- One teaspoon of garlic
- One teaspoon of cumin
- ¼ teaspoon of cinnamon

- ½ teaspoon of oregano
- One teaspoon salt
- 32 grams of boneless salmon

Instructions:

1. Mix all ingredients in a bowl and let marinate for at least 30 minutes.
2. Meanwhile preheat the grill to 350 F.
3. Place the salmon fillet on the hot grill and cook for 18 minutes or until it is well cooked.

NUTRITIONAL INFORMATION:

Calories per serving: 342; Carbohydrates: 1.5 g; Protein: 31.1 g; Fat: 22.7 g; Fiber: 0.3 g

❖ Coconut Shrimp:

Servings: 4

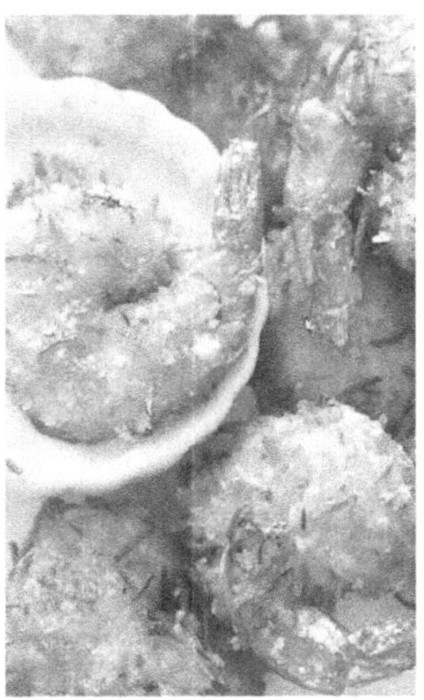

Ingredients:

- Two tablespoons rapeseed oil
- One large egg
- 2/3 tablespoon of water
- ¾ cups of dried coconut flakes
- ¾ teaspoon salt
- ½ teaspoon of black pepper

- 1 pound shell

Instructions:

1. Heat the oil in a frying pan over medium heat.
2. Mix the eggs and water in a bowl. Set aside.
3. Mix coconut flakes, salt and pepper in another bowl.
4. First, dip the shrimp with eggs and then with coconut.
5. Bake for 3 minutes or until golden brown.

NUTRITIONAL INFORMATION:
Calories per serving: 260; Carbohydrates: 2.5 g; Protein: 18.1 g; Fat : 19 g; Fiber: 0.9 g

❖ Fried Cod and Broccoli with Hazelnuts:

Servings: 1

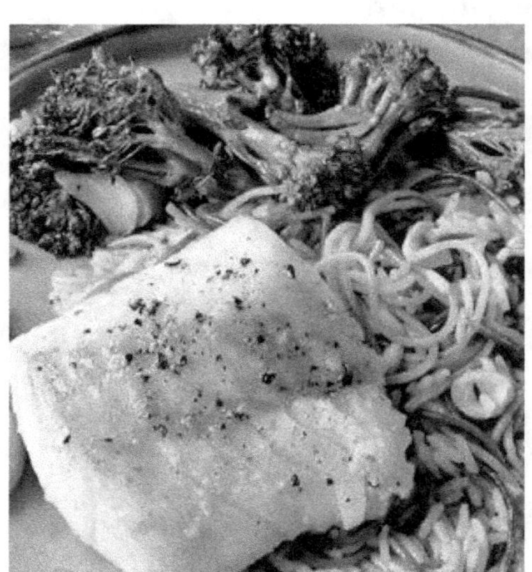

Ingredients:

- 6 grams of cod fillet
- 1 ½ cup chopped broccoli
- One tablespoon parsley
- One tablespoon butter
- Ten hazelnuts
- One slice of lemon

Instructions:

1. Preheat the oven to 350 F.
2. Make a foil bag and place the fish and broccoli in it.
3. Add the remaining ingredients.
4. Fold the aluminum bags and seal the edges by crimping them.
5. Put in the oven and cook for 15 minutes.

NUTRITIONAL INFORMATION:

Calories per serving: 495; Carbohydrates: 5.7 g; Protein: 36.8 g; Fat: 34.8 g; Fiber: 3.2 g

❖ Salad with Crab and Avocado:

Servings: 3

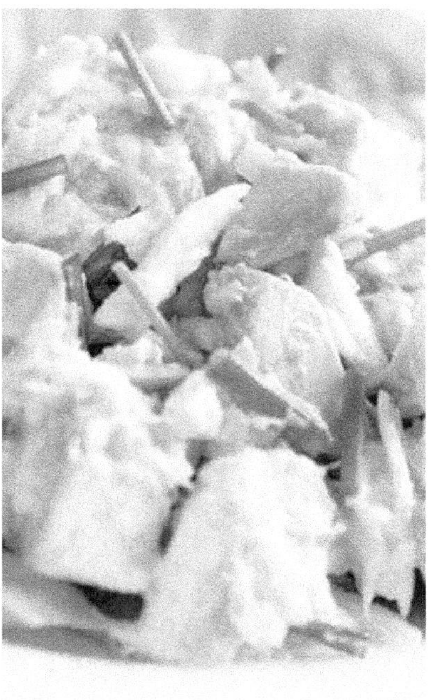

Ingredients:

- Three tablespoons organic egg mayonnaise
- Two tablespoons of freshly squeezed lemon juice
- One teaspoon of cumin
- ½ teaspoon of bell pepper

- 1 cup shredded crab
- 2 stalks of celery, finely chopped
- One avocado boneless, skinless and sliced
- 3 cups of chopped watercress

Instructions:

1. Combine mayonnaise, lime juice, caraway seeds and bell pepper in a large bowl.
2. Add crab meat and celery. Mix carefully to combine.
3. Add avocado slices and watercress.
4. Mix to combine.
5. Chill before serving, if you wish.

NUTRITIONAL INFORMATION:

Calories per serving: 255; Carbohydrates: 5.1 g; Protein: 24.7 g; Fat: 15.1 g; Fiber: 2.3 g

❖ Creole Shrimp Salad:

Servings: 5

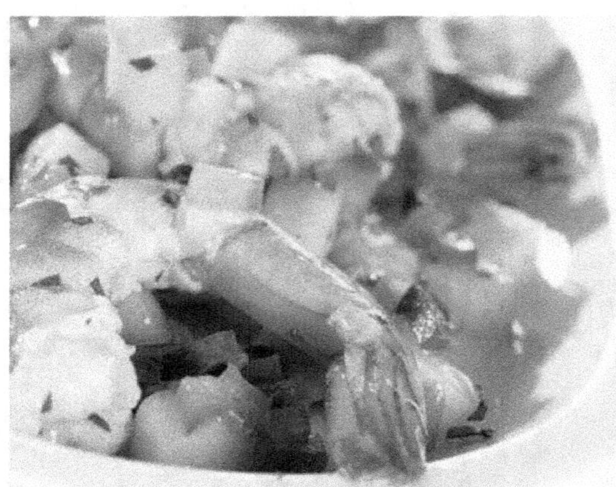

Ingredients:

- Two tablespoons of vegetable oil
- Two tablespoons of parsley
- One tablespoon grated radish spicy
- 1/3 teaspoon Tabasco sauce
- 2/3 tablespoons white wine vinegar

- Two teaspoons of Dijon mustard
- One teaspoon pepper
- ½ teaspoon of garlic
- ¼ teaspoon ground black pepper
- ½ teaspoon salt
- ½ stalk celery, finely chopped
- 2 pound cooked shrimp
- Two green onions, finely chopped

Instructions:

1. In a salad bowl, mix vegetable oil, parsley, horseradish, Tabasco sauce, white wine vinegar, Dijon mustard, bell pepper, and garlic.
2. Add celery, shrimp and spring onions.
3. Mix to combine all ingredients.
4. Cool before serving.

NUTRITIONAL INFORMATION:
calories per serving: 210; Carbohydrates: 0.6 g; Protein: 31 g; Fat: 7.4 g; Fiber: 0 g

❖ Curry Fish with Red Pepper:

Servings: 3

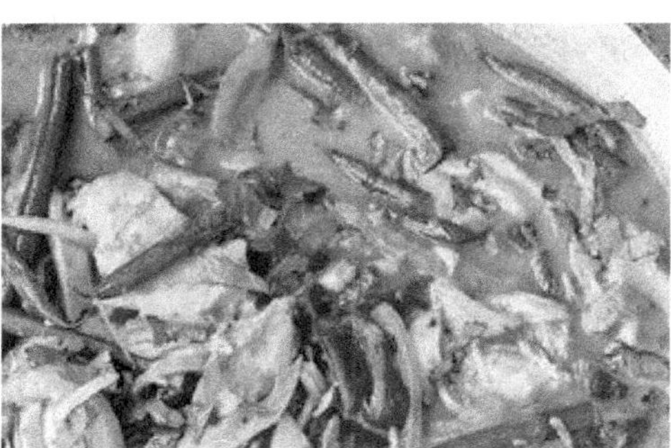

Ingredients:

- 1 ½ cup of coconut cream
- ½ tablespoon red chili paste
- Two teaspoons of ginger
- 1 ½ tablespoons fish sauce
- Three teaspoons of stevia sweetener
- 1 pound of white fish

- 3 cups of sweet red pepper, minced
- ½ ounce freshly squeezed lime juice

Instructions:

1. Heat the coconut oil in a large frying pan over medium heat and add the chili paste, ginger and fish sauce. Bring to boil before adding sweetener.
2. Add the fish fillet, bell pepper and lime juice.
3. Close the lid and cook for 10 minutes.
4. Season with salt and pepper.

NUTRITIONAL INFORMATION:
Calories per serving: 291; Carbohydrates: 3.1 g; Protein: 37.8 g; Fat: 12.3 g; Fibre: 0.9 g

Chapter fifteen: meat and vegetable intermittent fasting recipes

❖ **Asian Vegetable Bowl:**

Servings: 6

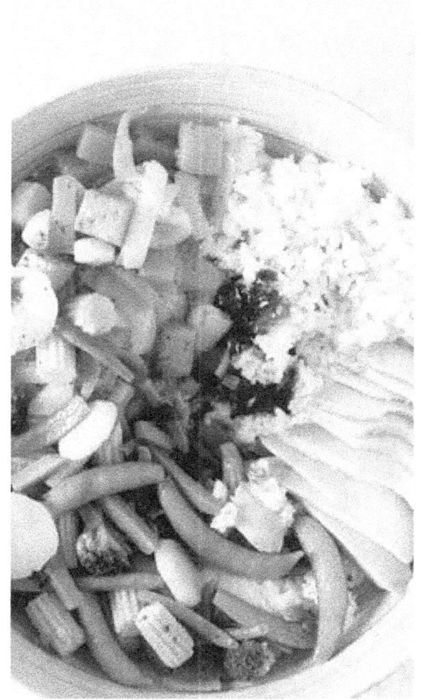

Ingredients:

- 6 cups chicken broth
- Four tablespoons soy sauce
- 2 cups cabbage
- 2 cups sliced mushrooms
- One garlic
- One serrano, chopped
- 3 cup chopped onions
- Three teaspoons grated ginger
- 1 cup chopped tomato
- 6 ounces, cubes
- ½ tablespoon coriander, minced

Instructions:

1. Boil the broth and soy sauce in a pan over medium heat.
2. Once the stock is boiling, reduce the heat and add cabbage, mushrooms, garlic and serrano pepper.
3. Add green onions, ginger, tomato and tofu.
4. Close the lid and cook for 5 minutes.
5. Add coriander before serving.

NUTRITIONAL INFORMATION:
calories per serving: 65; Carbohydrates: 1.8 g; Protein : 6.7 g; Fat: 2.1 g; Fibre: 0 g

❖ Fried Tofu with Asian Marinade:

Servings: 2

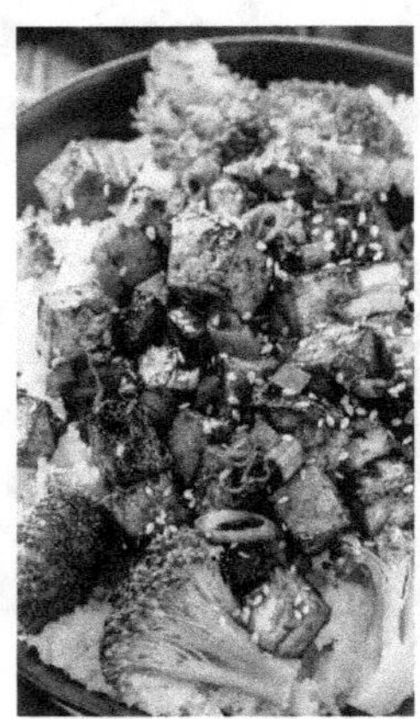

Ingredients:

- Two tablespoons of soy sauce
- One tablespoon olive oil
- ½ teaspoon of sesame oil
- One tablespoon ginger
- One garlic
- ½ tablespoon sugar
- One tablespoon white vinegar
- 6 ounces firm tofu, sliced

Instructions:

1. Mix all ingredients except tofu in a bowl. Mix until well mixed.
2. Marinate the tofu slices for at least 2 hours.
3. Preheat the oven to 375 F.
4. Place the tofu slices on a greased baking sheet.
5. Bake for 15 minutes or until golden brown and crispy.

NUTRITIONAL INFORMATION:
Calories per serving: 232; Carbohydrates: 4.8 g; Protein: 17.7 g;
Fat: 14.9 g; Fiber : 3.3 g

❖ Fried Tofu with Chipotle Marinade:

Servings: 2

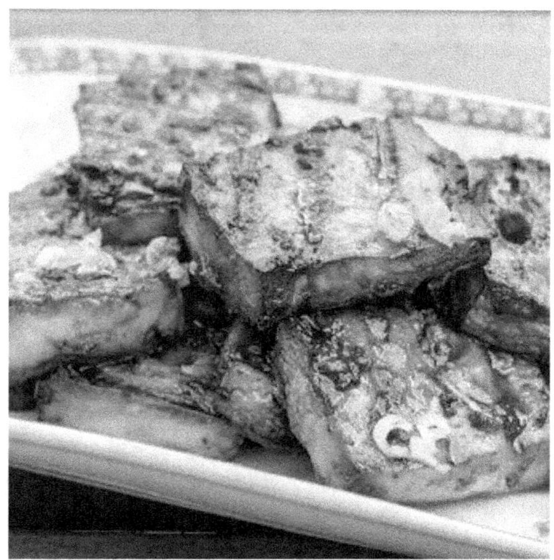

Ingredients:

- 6 ounces firm tofu, sliced
- One cut kIp , sliced
- ½ cup mayonnaise
- 1/3 cup regular Greek yoghurt
- ¼ cups of coriander, chopped
- ¼ teaspoon of cumin
- ¼ teaspoon of dried dill
- Salt to taste

Instructions:

1. Marinate tofu with the rest of the ingredients for a minimum of
2 hours.
2. Preheat the oven to 375 F.
3. Place the tofu slices on a greased baking sheet.

4. Bake for 15 minutes or until golden brown and crispy.

NUTRITIONAL INFORMATION:
Calories per serving: 227; Carbohydrates: 1 g; Protein: 15.8 g; Fat: 15.9 g; Fiber: 0 g

❖ **Spinach and Blackberry Salad with Goat Cheese Medallions :**

Servings: 5

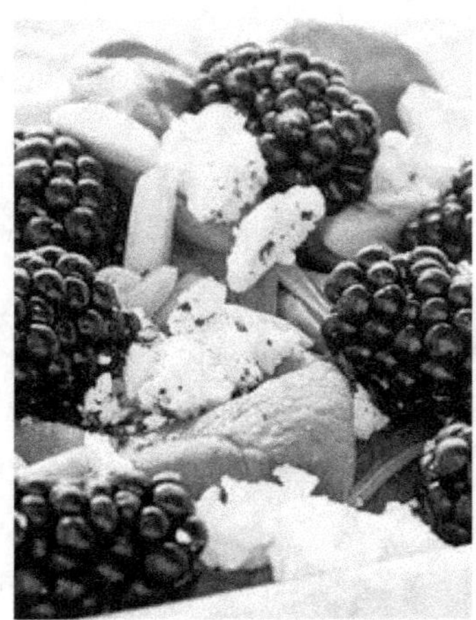

Ingredients:

- goat cheese rolled 6 grams in balls
- One large egg, beaten
- ¼ cup chopped walnuts
- Two tablespoons olive oil
- ¼ onion, chopped
- ¾ teaspoon of cinnamon
- 12 grams of blackberries
- 1/3 tablespoons balsamic vinegar
- 9 cups baby spinach, washed and cut
- 30 cherry tomatoes

Instructions:

1. Preheat the oven to 375 F.
2. Dip the goat cheese balls into beaten eggs and roll the chopped nuts. Place the round cheese balls on a baking sheet and bake for

10 minutes. When this is done, remove it from the oven and set it aside.

3. Heat olive oil in a pan and fry the onion and cinnamon fragrant. Add blackberries and use a fork to crush the berries. Keep stirring for 3 minutes and then add the balsamic vinegar. Set aside and let cool.

4. Add baked cheese medallions, spinach and tomatoes to the salad bowl. Pour cooled blackberry sauce.

NUTRITIONAL INFORMATION:
Calories per serving: 222; Carbohydrates: 8.2 g; Protein: 9. 2 g; Fat: 14.9 g; Fiber: 3.4 g

❖ Hot Cauliflower Buffalo:

Servings: 4

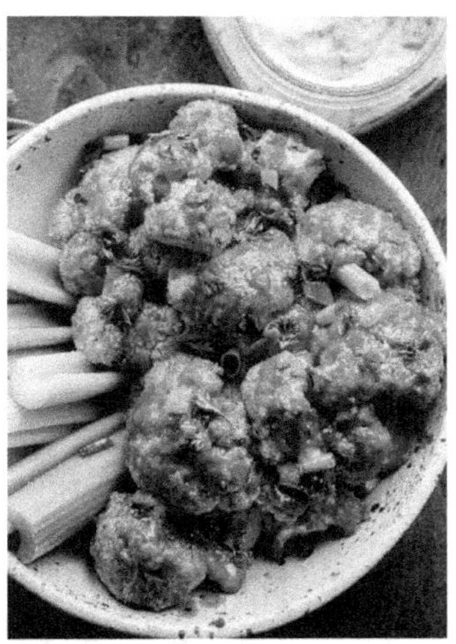

Ingredients:

- One cauliflower flower cut into inflorescences
- Two tablespoons olive oil
- Four tablespoons chicken wing sauce
- Three teaspoons of Sriracha hot sauce
- Two tablespoons unsalted butter
- 1 ½ ounce blue cheese

Instructions:

1. Preheat the oven to 375 F.
2. Sprinkle cauliflower flowers with olive oil. Place on a baking sheet and bake in the oven for 40 minutes.
3. While the baked florets are cooking, prepare the sauce by combining the wings sauce, hot Sriracha sauce, unsalted butter and blue cheese.   4. Once the cauliflower has been baked, pour the sauce and mix to coat.
5. Serve hot.

NUTRITIONAL INFORMATION:
Calories per serving: 177; Carbohydrates: 4.2 g; Protein: 5.3 g; Fat: 14.9 g; Fiber: 1.8 g

❖ **Casserole with Swiss Chard and Cheese:**

Servings: 2

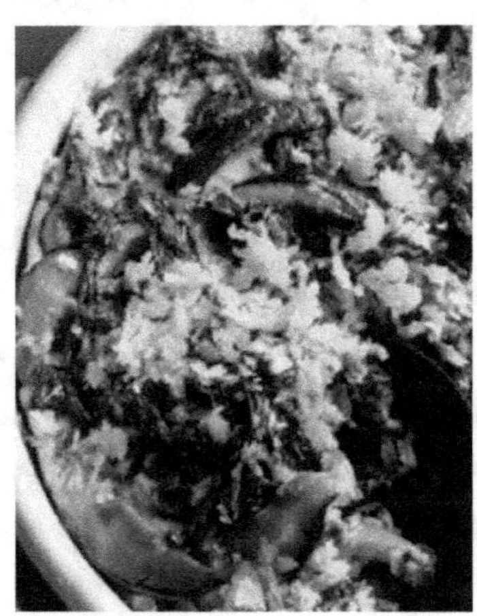

Ingredients:

- Two tablespoons olive oil
- ¾ pounds chard, coil and trim
- One sweet red pepper, minced
- One onion, chopped
- ½ teaspoon salt
- ¼ teaspoon of black pepper
- 1 ½ cups Munster cheese

- ½ cup of grated Parmesan cheese

Instructions:

1. Preheat the oven to 375 F.
2. In a pan, heat one tablespoon of olive oil and fry the chard for 3 minutes on high heat until it dries. Pour on a sieve and press to remove excess moisture.
3. Heat the remaining olive oil in a pan and fry the peppers and onions until they are fragrant and transparent. Add the chard and season with salt and pepper.
4. Put the vegetables in a baking dish and sprinkle with both types of cheese.
5. Bake for 10 minutes.

NUTRITIONAL INFORMATION:
Calories per serving: 195; Carbohydrates: 1.6 g; Protein: 10.6 g; Fat: 15.3 g; Fiber: 0.5 g

❖ Cobb Salad:

Servings: 2

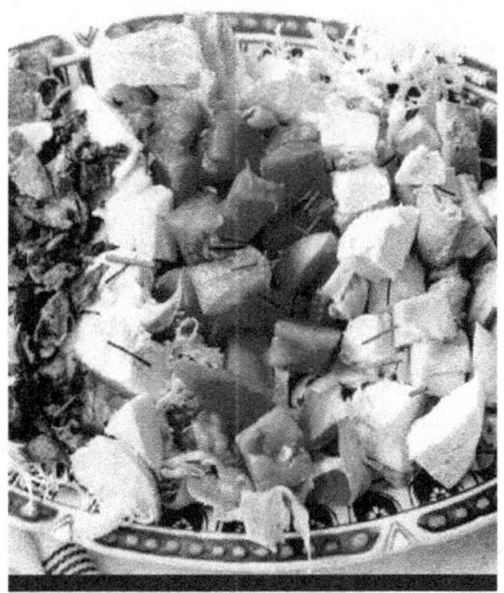

Ingredients:

- ½ cup romaine lettuce washed
- ½ cup iceberg lettuce washed
- Eight slices of bacon, fried until crispy

- 16 ounces cooked, shredded chicken
- Five cherry tomatoes
- Four green onions, finely chopped
- Four tablespoons wine vinegar
- One teaspoon of mustard Dijon
- ½ cup olive oil
- One avocado butter, peeled and chopped
- One boiled egg, peeled and sliced
- 6 oz blue cheese

Instructions:

1. In a bowl, mix romaine lettuce and iceberg lettuce, bacon, chicken, tomatoes, and green onions.
2. Mix the vinegar, mustard and olive oil in another bowl.
3. Pour the salad.
4. Place the slices of avocado and eggs on top.
5. Sprinkle with grated blue cheese.

NUTRITIONAL INFORMATION:

Calories per serving: 600; Carbohydrates: 3.4 g; Protein: 35.8 g; Fat: 48.3 g; Fiber: 1.4 g

❖ **Coconut and Curry Tempeh:**

Servings: 4

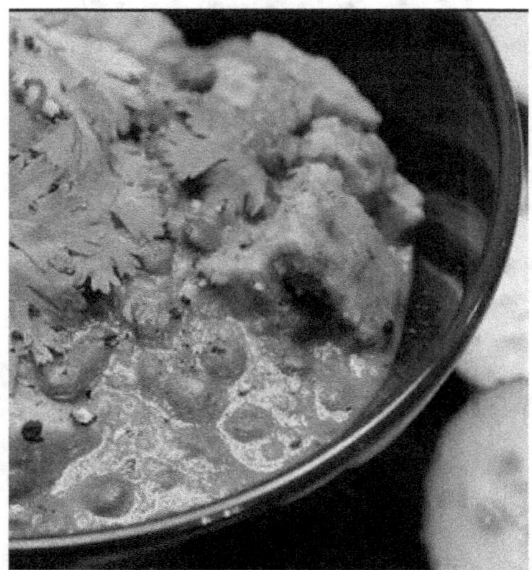

Ingredients:

- ¼ cup of water
- 2/3 tablespoons of soy sauce
- Two tablespoons sesame oil
- 16 ounces tempeh
- ½ cup chopped onion
- One tablespoon ginger
- 3/4 cup coconut milk
- ½ tablespoon freshly squeezed lime juice
- One tablespoon of natural peanut butter
- Two teaspoons of curry powder
- ½ teaspoon of cumin
- ¼ teaspoon of cayenne pepper
- ¼ teaspoon salt
- coriander 1-ounce cut

Instructions:

1. Put water, one tablespoon of soy sauce and one teaspoon of sesame oil in a baking dish. Add the tempeh and marinate for 30 minutes.
2. In a large skillet warm sesame oil and fried onions and ginger in the remaining oil until the aroma appears.
3. Add the pickled pace and cook for 5 minutes on each side.
4. Meanwhile, add coconut and curry sauce, coconut oil, lime juice, peanut butter, curry powder, cumin, cayenne pepper and salt.
5. Pour tempeh sauce and cook for 5 minutes.
6. Lower the heat and cook for 10 minutes.
7. Garnish with chopped coriander.

NUTRITIONAL INFORMATION:

Calories per serving: 511; Carbohydrates: 1.2 g; Protein: 25.5 g; Fat: 41.9 g; Fiber: 1 g

❖ Creamy Mushroom Soup:

Servings: 3

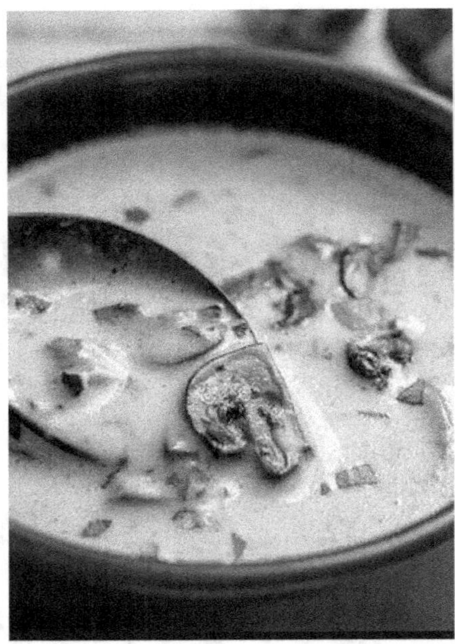

Ingredients:

- One teaspoon dried thyme
- Two tins of chicken broth with a low sodium content
- ½ cup of water
- 20 ounces chopped mushrooms
- 1 cup of fat cream
- Salt and pepper to taste
- One tablespoon freshly squeezed lemon juice

Instructions:

1. Heat olive oil in a large saucepan over medium heat.
2. Bake onion and thyme until fragrant.
3. Add chicken broth, water and mushrooms. Close the lid and cook.
4. After cooking, lower the heat and cook for 10 minutes.
5. Remove from heat and add cream.
6. Transfer to a blender and crush until smooth. Return to the pan and season with salt and pepper.
7. Add lemon juice at the end.

NUTRITIONAL INFORMATION:

Calories per serving: 158; Carbohydrates: 0.8 g; Protein: 3.5 g ; Fat: 15 g Fiber: 0 g

❖ Eggplant and Napoleonic Goat Cheese :

Servings: 4

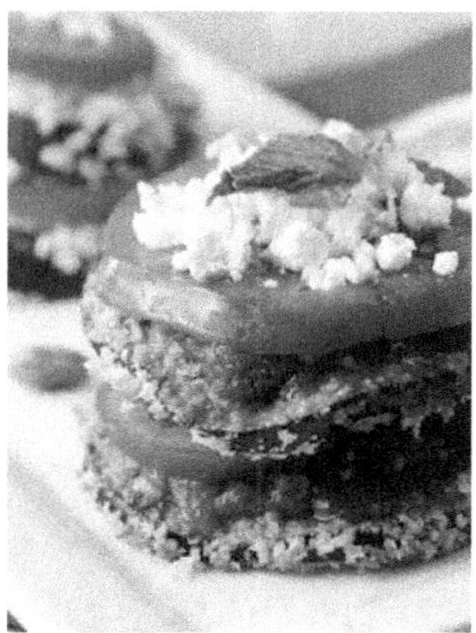

Ingredients:

- 1 pound of chopped eggplant
- ¾ teaspoon salt
- Four tablespoons olive oil
- ½ teaspoon of black pepper
- 20 asparagus spears
- 5½ grams of goat cheese, sliced
- One teaspoon dried thyme
- Four tablespoons unsweetened ketchup
- Two tablespoons water
- ½ teaspoon of oregano
- ¼ teaspoon rosemary

Instructions:

1. Heat the grill over medium heat. Prepare a baking tray with paper towels.
2. Spray eggplant with salt and two tablespoons of olive oil. Add black pepper. Mix to coat and bake.
3. Spread the asparagus with the remaining olive oil and fry with the eggplant.

4. Transfer the vegetables to the baking tray lined with paper towels.
5. Arrange asparagus, aubergines and cheese. Set aside.
6. Mix the rest of the ingredients in a bowl. Beat and pour over vegetables.

NUTRITIONAL INFORMATION:
calories per serving: 316; Carbohydrates: 6 g; Protein: 11.6 g; Fat: 25.9 g; Fiber: 3.5 g

❖ **Eggplant Rollatini:**

Servings: 3

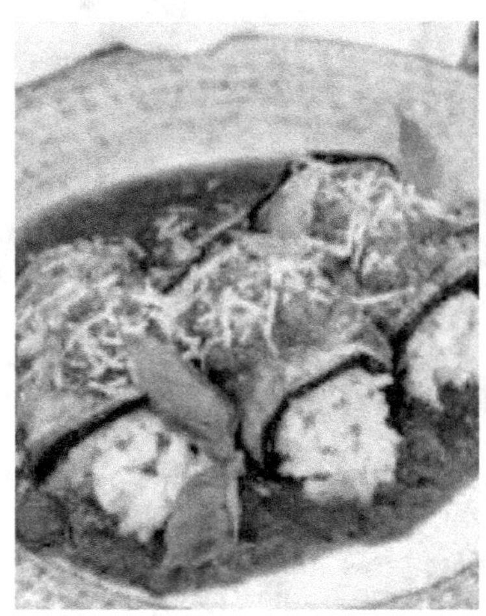

Ingredients:

- Three slices of eggplant
- 1 ½ cup of water
- ¾ cup of chickpea flour
- four large eggs
- ¼ cups olive oil
- 1 cup ketchup
- ¼ cup ricotta
- 1/3 cup Parmesan cheese
- 4 slices of mozzarella cheese
- ¼ teaspoon salt
- ¼ teaspoon of black pepper
- ¼ cup parsley

Instructions:

1. Season the eggplant with salt. Place in a filter and press to remove excess water. Then rinse and dry. Set aside.
2. In another bowl, mix water, chickpea flour and two eggs until blended.
3. Dip the eggplant in the dough and place on a baking sheet with extra virgin olive oil. Bake for 3 minutes until golden. Place on a plate laid with kitchen paper and set aside.
4. Preheat the oven to 400 F.
5. Place the eggplant layers on the bottom in the baking dish. Pour in the tomato sauce. Sprinkle with ricotta, parmesan cheese and mozzarella.
6. Season with salt and pepper. Garnish with parsley.
7. Bake for 10 minutes.

NUTRITIONAL INFORMATION:
Calories per serving: 433; Carbohydrates: 5.7 g; Protein: 24.7 g; Fat: 31.1 g; Fiber: 2.4 g

❖ **Curry Cauliflower Soup:**

Servings: 4

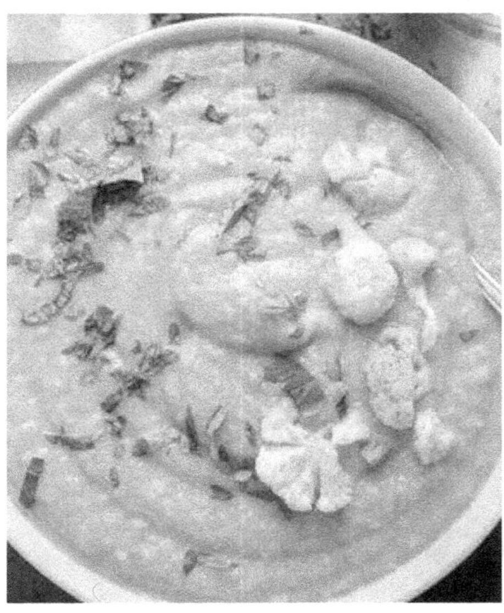

Ingredients:

- One tablespoon olive oil
- One onion
- Two cloves garlic, finely chopped
- One tablespoon curry powder
- One teaspoon of ginger
- One cauliflower, cut into flowers
- One can of chicken broth with little sodium
- 2 cups of water
- 1 cup of fat cream
- 2 tbsp chopped onion

Instructions:

1. Heat the olive oil in a large pan.
2. Fry onion and garlic until fragrant. Add curry powder and ginger and cook for 1 minute.
3. Add the cauliflower flowers, broth and water. Boil over high heat.
4. Reduce the heat to a minimum and cook for 20 minutes.
5. Once the cauliflower inflorescences become soft, add cream.
6. Go to the blender and blend until smooth.
7. Put the mixture back into the pot and garnish with onions.
8. Add salt and pepper to taste.

NUTRITIONAL INFORMATION:
Calories per serving: 198; Carbohydrates: 2.7 g; Protein: 3.5 g; Fat: 17.7 g; Fiber: 0.3 g

❖ **Irish Pub Salad:**

Servings: 6

Ingredients:

- 9 cups of chopped butter
- 2 cups shredded red cabbage
- Three stalks of celery, finely chopped
- 1 cup cauliflower stem, cut into inflorescences
- Eight fried mushrooms, sliced

- ½ cup chopped cucumber
- ½ cup chopped zucchini
- Ten cherry tomatoes
- Six large hard-boiled eggs
- 6 grams Roquefort cheese
- 2/3 cup egg mayonnaise
- ¼ cups of thick cream
- ¼ cup of water
- 1/8 teaspoon of black pepper
- ¼ teaspoon salt
- 1 ½ teaspoon rosemary
- 1/8 teaspoon tarragon

Instructions:

1. In a bowl, mix salad, cabbage, celery, cauliflower, mushrooms, cucumbers, zucchini, tomatoes, eggs, and cheese.
2. In another bowl, mix mayonnaise, cream, water, black pepper, salt, rosemary, and tarragon.
3. Pour the salad. Mix to combine.

NUTRITIONAL INFORMATION:
Calories per serving: 433; Carbohydrates: 3.1 g; Protein: 15.4 g; Fat: 37.1 g; Fiber: 1.9 g

❖ **Italian Pasta and Bean Soup:**

Servings: 4

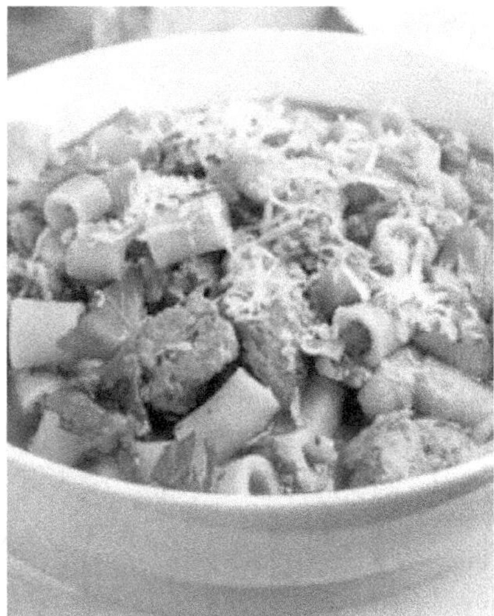

Ingredients:

- Two tablespoons olive oil
- 1 cup of grated Parmesan cheese
- One stalk of celery, finely chopped
- One small chopped carrot
- ½ onions
- 1/3 cup freshly cooked ham
- Two teaspoons of garlic
- A cup of tomato cubes
- Three cans of chicken broth
- Three teaspoons of oregano
- 1 cup of cannellini beans, rinse and drain
- ¾ cups of whole-grain penne
- One tablespoon chopped parsley

Instructions:

1. Heat the oil in a pan over high heat. Bake celery, carrots, onions and ham for 5 minutes.
2. Add the garlic and fry for 30 seconds. Add tomatoes, chicken broth, oregano and cannellini beans. Stir a cent.
3. Bring to the boil and cook for 20 minutes.
4. Garnish with parsley.

NUTRITIONAL INFORMATION:
Calories per serving: 210; Carbohydrates: 6.9 g; Protein: 14.1 g; Fat: 10.5 g; Fiber: 3.7 g

❖ **Eggplant Lasagna:**

Servings: 6

Ingredients:

- 1 ½ pound of eggplant, cut lengthwise
- ¼ pound ground beef
- 1 cup ketchup
- 4 portobello mushrooms (stems are cut and removed)
- Salt and pepper to taste

- 2 cups ricotta cheese
- Two large eggs
- ¼ cup of Parmesan cheese
- One packet of chopped spinach
- 1 pound mozzarella cheese

Instructions:

1. Salt the eggplant slices in a colander. Click to remove the fluid. Rinse, dry and reserve.
2. Put the minced meat in a medium-sized pan and cook over medium heat. Beat the meat with a spoon. Bake for 6 minutes until golden. Add tomato sauce and reserve.
3. Boil the mushrooms in a pan and season with salt and pepper. Set aside.
4. Put ricotta cheese, eggs and parmesan cheese in a blender.
5. Collect lasagna by placing eggplant in a baking dish. Put spinach on top, then a mixture of meat and tomatoes and a mixture of cheese. Repeat the layers until all components have been placed in the baking dish.
6. Bake in a preheated oven at 400 F for 20 minutes.

NUTRITIONAL INFORMATION:
Calories per serving: 358; Carbohydrates: 3.4 g; Protein: 24.1 g; Fat: 25.8 g; Fiber: 2.5 g

❖ Goat Cheese Marinated with Citrus Basil:

Servings: 4

Ingredients:

- ½ cup olive oil
- ½ teaspoon of garlic, finely chopped
- 4 tablespoons chopped basil
- One tablespoon grated lemon zest
- 1/8 freshly squeezed lime juice
- ½ teaspoon of whole black pepper
- 12 ounces goat cheese, sliced

Instructions:

1. Combine all ingredients except chopped goat cheese.
2. Put slices of goat cheese in a baking dish and pour the sauce over it.
3. Serve cold.

NUTRITIONAL INFORMATION:
calories per serving: 176; Carbohydrates: 0.1 g; Protein: 5.7 g; Fat: 17.1 g; Fiber: 0 g

❖ **Helmet Flower Risotto:**

Servings: 4

Ingredients:

- 2 cups chopped cauliflower
- One tablespoon olive oil
- One tablespoon chopped shallots
- ½ cup vegetable broth
- Two tablespoons thick cream
- 2 tablespoons chopped parsley
- ½ cup of Parmesan cheese

Instructions:

1. Place the cauliflower flowers in the food processor. Pulsate to the size of the beans.
2. Heat the oil in a frying pan over medium-high heat and fry the shallots until soft.
3. Add the cauliflower and stir to cover with olive oil. Add the vegetable stock and let cook until they soften.
4. Add cream, parsley and cheese. Keep cooking for 3 minutes.

NUTRITIONAL INFORMATION:
Calories per serving: 117; Carbohydrates: 1.3 g; Protein: 5.1 g; Fat: 9.3 g; Fiber: 0.9 g

❖ **Fried Cauliflower and Green Beans with Oyster Sauce:**

Servings: 4

Ingredients:

- 1 pound of cooked cauliflower, cut into flowers
- Two tablespoons of soy sauce
- One teaspoon of honey
- Two tablespoons of vegetable oil
- Two teaspoons of ginger
- ½ teaspoon of garlic
- 4 grams of green beans, sliced
- ¼ cup of water
- Two tablespoons oyster sauce
- 1 oz almonds
- Three medium-sized onions, finely chopped

Instructions:

1. Put the cauliflower in a bowl and add soy sauce and honey. Mix to coat.
2. Heat vegetable oil in a pan and fry ginger and garlic until fragrant.
3. Bake marinated cauliflower and beans.
4. Add water and season with oyster sauce.
5. Bake for 8 minutes or until soft.
6. Garnish with almonds and onions.

NUTRITIONAL INFORMATION:
Calories per serving: 94; Carbohydrates: 3 g; Protein: 3.5 g; Fat: 6.1 g; Fiber: 2.3 g

❖ Mac Cauliflower and Cheese:

Servings: 4

Ingredients:

- 1 cup cooked cauliflower, chopped, and dried
- 1 cup of fat cream
- 2 ounces cream cheese
- 1 ½ teaspoon of mustard

- 1 ½ cup grated cheddar cheese
- One clove garlic
- Salt and pepper to taste
- ¼ the teaspoon sauce (optional)

Instructions:

1. Preheat the oven to 375 F.
2. Put all the ingredients in the bowl. Mix to cover all ingredients with sauce.
3. Put in a baking dish and bake for 15 minutes.

NUYTRITIONAL INFORMATION:
Calories per serving: 320; Carbohydrates: 3.6 g; Protein: 11.4 g; Fat: 27.5 g; Fiber: 1.8 g

❖ **Caponata:**

Servings: 1

ingredients:

- ¼ cups of olive oil
- 12 ounces eggplant
- ½ red onion, chopped
- ½ teaspoon of chopped garlic
- ½ large pepper
- ¼ cup of water
- Two tablespoons of parsley
- One teaspoon salt
- Two tablespoons capers, drained
- Two tablespoons of freshly squeezed lemon juice

Instructions:

1. Heat the olive oil in a saucepan over medium heat.
2. Add eggplant, onion, garlic and pepper.
3. Add water and boil.
4. Cover and simmer until the aubergines are soft.
5. Add parsley, salt, capers and lemon juice.

NUTRITIONAL INFORMATION:

Calories per serving: 101; Carbohydrates: 2.3 g; Protein: 0.9 g; Fat: 9.5 g Fiber: 0.8 g

❖ Breakfast Meat Burgers:

Servings: 6

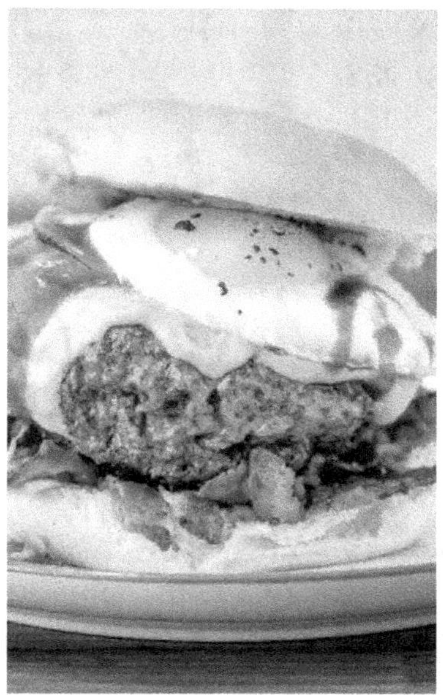

Ingredients:

- Two teaspoons basil
- One teaspoon garlic, finely chopped
- Two tablespoons almond flour
- Three sun-dried tomatoes, finely chopped
- ½ cup of ground sausage
- Eight slices of cooked bacon
- Five eggs
- 1 pound of ground pork

Instructions:

1. Combine meat and one egg in a bowl.
2. Add the sun-dried tomatoes, garlic, almond flour and basil.
3. Shape the meat burgers with your hands and reserve.
4. Cook the bacon in a pan and set aside.

5. In the same pan, cook each side for five minutes until cooked.

6. Bake the sausage and set aside.
7. Bake four eggs separately and set aside.
8. Assemble a breakfast burger by laying an empanada with sausage and eggs.

NUTRITIONAL INFORMATION:
calories per serving: 653; Carbohydrates: 19.6 g; Protein: 71.3 g; Fat: 56.8 g; Fiber: 6 g

❖ **Slow Pork:**

Servings: 6

ingredients:

- Six boneless pork chops
- Two cans cream chicken soup
- 1 cup of fat cream
- 1 of ranch salad dressing
- Salt and pepper to taste
- Parsley sprig

Instructions:

1. Place the pork tenderloin in a slow cooker and add the chicken soup.
2. Cook over medium heat for 30 minutes.
3. Add thick cream and ranch dressing.
4. Cook another 5 minutes.
5. Season with salt and pepper.
6. Garnish with a sprig of parsley.

NUTRITIONAL INFORMATION:
calories per serving: 448; Carbohydrates: 9.4 g; Protein: 44.3 g; Fat: 24 g; Fiber: 0.2 g

❖ **Italian Stewed Lamb:**

Servings: 8

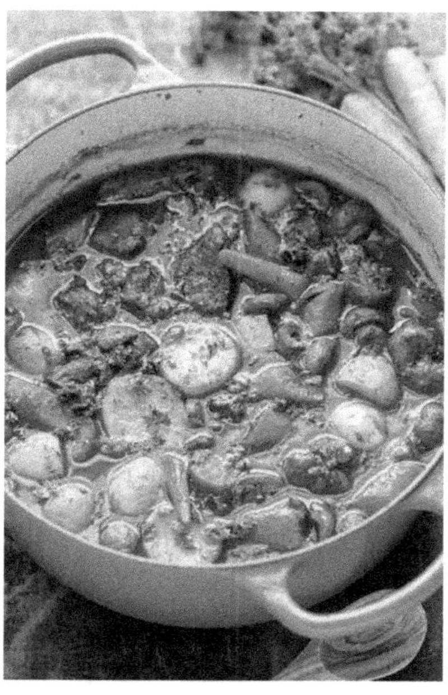

Ingredients:

- ¼ cup of olive oil
- 3.5 pounds of boneless lamb leg
- 6 finely chopped garlic cloves
- two tablespoons Italian herbs
- ½ cup of lemon juice
- 5 cups of water
- Salt and pepper to taste

Instructions:

1. Heat the oil in a medium-sized pan.
2. Bake the leg of lamb until all sides are golden brown.
3. Put in a pan and add garlic, Italian herbs and lime juice.
4. Pour 5 cups of water and season with salt and pepper.
5. Pour in oil, garlic, Italian herbs and lemon juice.
6. Stir to mix all ingredients.
7. Close the lid and cook for 4 hours.

NUTRITIONAL INFORMATION:

Calories per serving: 339; Carbohydrates: 3.04 g; Protein: 40.4 g; Fat: 17.3 g ; Fiber: 0.4 g

Chapter sixteen: Conclusion

First of all, I want to thank you for taking this path of knowledge and for reaching the end of this book. Congratulations on saying NO to ill health, stubborn weight gain, depression, dementia and premature ageing, and a loud NO to the idea that we cannot naturally heal our bodies and minds! When I first sat down to write this guide to understand and use the secrets of intermittent fasting, to people like you: those who are not satisfied with the current state of affairs, which they had been told and did not do that. They are ready to let go of their desire for good health, vitality, physical fitness, clarity of mind and longevity just because conventional medicine and nutrition tells them that this is impossible. If you already have started intermittent fasting, i.e., there is no doubt it began with the *look* and feel *of* the fantastic effects which I have covered in this book. Continuing your journey to achieve liveliness and well-being for life, remember that you are travelling through an old, proven form of prosperity. I urge you to use this as a guide. When people ask about the use of intermittent fasting, you will not only be able to point to visible changes in your body, appearance and energy levels, but you have all the scientific evidence at hand to prove that the old method works! Live and heal! These days it works just as well as centuries ago! Finally, I wish you all the best on your journey to restore, rejuvenate and protect every cell in your body and mind. I would like to remind you to view the index of recipes at the end of this book for a selection of delicious dishes. This is handy for use with different types of intermittent fasting, which we cover in this guide! Good luck and good health!

www.ingramcontent.com/pod-product-compliance
Lightning Source LLC
Chambersburg PA
CBHW070715250726
48662CB00001B/435